BASIC URINALYSIS

BASIC URINALYSIS

George J. Race, M.D., Ph.D.
Professor of Pathology, Associate Dean for Continuing Education, The University of Texas Health Science Center at Dallas Southwestern Medical School; Pathologist-in-Chief, Department of Pathology, Dean of the A. Webb Roberts Center for Continuing Education in the Health Sciences, Baylor University Medical Center, Dallas, Texas

Martin G. White, M.D.
Director, Nephrology Division and Nephrology Laboratory, Baylor University Medical Center; Assistant Clinical Professor, Department of Internal Medicine, The University of Texas Health Science Center at Dallas Southwestern Medical School, Dallas, Texas.

With 16 Color Illustrations

Medical Department
Harper & Row, Publishers
Hagerstown, Maryland
New York, San Francisco, London

The authors and publisher have exerted every effort to ensure that drug selection and dosage set forth in this text are in accord with current recommendations and practice at the time of publication. However, in view of ongoing research, changes in government regulations, and the constant flow of information relating to drug therapy and drug reactions, the reader is urged to check the package insert for each drug for any change in indications and dosage and for added warnings and precautions. This is particularly important when the recommended agent is a new and/or infrequently employed drug.

79-80-81-82-83-84—10-9-8-7-6-5-4-3-2-1

BASIC URINALYSIS. Copyright © 1979 by Harper & Row, Publishers, Inc. All rights reserved. No part of this book may be used or reproduced in any manner whatsoever without written permission except in the case of brief quotations embodied in critical articles and reviews. Printed in the United States of America. For information address Medical Department, Harper & Row, Publishers, Inc., 2350 Virginia Avenue, Hagerstown, Maryland 21740.

Library of Congress Cataloging in Publication Data

Race, George J
  Basic Urinalysis.
  Bibliography: p.
  Includes index.
  1. Urine—Analysis. I. White, Martin G., 1939-joint author. II. Title.
[DNLM: 1. Urine—Analysis. QY185 R118b]
RB53.R32   616.07′566   78-11725
ISBN 0-06-142229-0

Dedicated to great teachers of pathologic physiology who have enlightened and stimulated us, especially Tinsley Harrison, M.D. (deceased), George Thorn, M.D., and Donald Seldin, M.D.

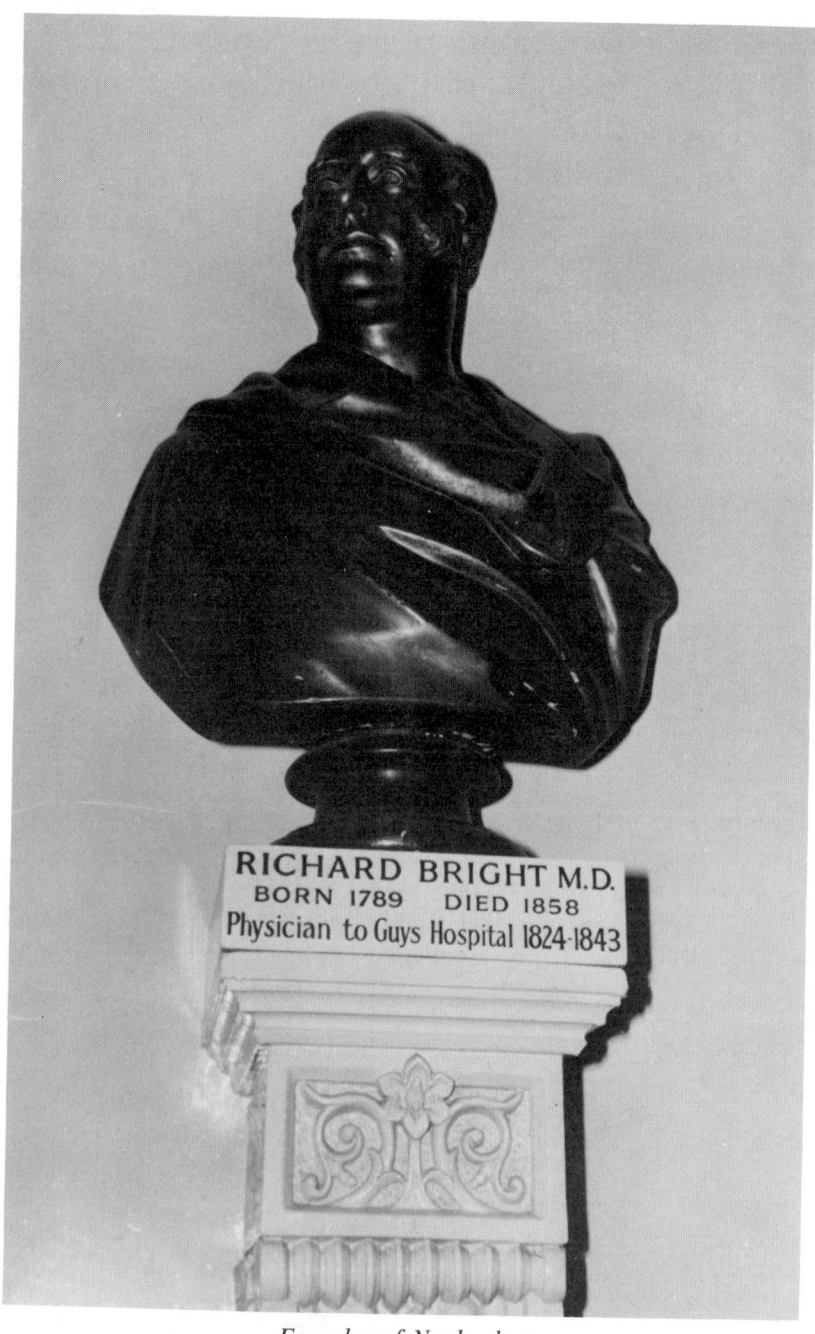

Founder of Nephrology

CONTENTS

PREFACE   *ix*

PART I   INTRODUCTION   *1*
1. History and Purpose of Urinalysis   *1*
2. Specimen Collection and Preservation   *7*

PART II   TESTING PROCEDURES   *12*
3. Physical Characteristics   *12*
4. Specific Gravity and Osmolality   *14*
5. Microscopic Examination   *18*
6. Clinical Screening   *27*
7. Urinary pH   *30*
8. Glucose and Other Sugars   *31*
9. Ketones   *34*
10. Protein   *37*
11. Addis Count   *48*
12. Urinary Pigments   *50*
13. Urine Fat   *64*
14. Calcium   *65*
15. Generalized Metabolic Derangements   *67*
16. Screening for Diseases, Drugs, or Poisons   *82*
17. Functional Tests   *87*

PART III   LABORATORY OPERATION   *101*
18. Automation of Urinalysis   *101*
19. Quality Control   *102*

REFERENCES   *105*
INDEX   *109*

PREFACE

Homer Smith once stated that the kidney is the most "intelligent" and important organ in the body. It is capable of discriminating internal environmental needs, regulating electrolytes and water, and establishing the thresholds for retention of needed products such as sugar and for excretion of unwanted products such as urea. The kidney has the ability to regulate blood pressure, to regulate blood volume, and to reciprocate with the adrenal cortex in the performance of biochemical jobs ranging from pH balance to osmotic pressure adjustment. Further, the kidney's ready production of excreted fluid makes it the ideal organ for indirect examination of the internal environment by studying its products of excretion. The kidney mirrors the physiologic status of the whole body.

The history of urinalysis is a study unto itself and makes most interesting reading. In the past, interpretation of abnormalities of urine by taste, color, smell, and turbidity was used. Sweet-tasting urine represented diabetes. Black urine might represent malarial hemolysis, and be indicative of a grave prognosis in black water fever.

The purpose of this small volume is to produce a readable, practical manual for the medical student, the physician desiring a short review, and the medical technologist faced with the daily operation of the urinalysis laboratory. It will tell the reader in a concise manner the nature of a procedure, methods for performance, and something of its significance and interpretation. Primarily, the book is written to bring together a great number of loose ends in common usage in medical laboratories. The information is not intended for research use but is presented for practical usage. Every clinical laboratory, large or small, relies heavily on its urinalysis section and places a great responsibility on this area because of its important contribution in both routine and diagnostic screening procedures. Throughout the text, "mg/dl" replaces "mg/percent" in conformance with current terminology.

A major portion of the material in this book represents an original contribution by Dr. E. E. Baird, Professor of Clinical Pathology and Director of the Clinical Laboratories, Department of Pathology of the University of Texas Medical Branch in Galveston, Texas. Dr. Baird's contribution was published in Harper & Row's four-volume series, LABORATORY MEDICINE, edited by G. J. Race, as Chapter 1, "Urinalysis," in Volume 4. A second important source is the teaching manual for the Urinalysis Laboratory, Department of Pathology, Baylor University Medical Center, Dallas, Texas. This manual was assembled under the general direction of Mr. Johnny Sills, Chief Medical Technologist, who was assisted by innumerable medical technologists, associates, students, and pathology residents through the years. We are grateful to Dr. Mary D. Bradley for the use of her material related to pediatric screening for disease. It is not possible to name each individual who made a contribution, but we wish to thank each person who worked diligently to make the material available. The Department of Laboratories of Baylor University Medical Center has supported this project with secretarial assistance, with photographic assistance by Mr. George Bridges and Dr. James L. Martin of the Electron Microscopy Laboratory, and by other means.

We are especially grateful to Dr. Joel Young, Dr. Norman Helgeson, Dr. Robert Speer, Dr. J. L. Matthews, Dr. G. V. K. Rao, and Mr. Johnny L. Sills, who reviewed and critiqued individual sections of the manuscript.

Finally, manuscript preparation and typing have required the assistance of several persons, especially Lee Rhea Capote, Beverly Gay, Linda Lewis, Nina Duncan, and Linda O'Rear. Rose Kraft, our editorial assistant, has taken major responsibility for all phases of preparation. Geneva Straughan has prepared and edited the final manuscript. Our special thanks goes to them.

Dallas, Texas
G.J.R.
M.G.W.

BASIC URINALYSIS

PART **1** INTRODUCTION

1 History and Purpose of Urinalysis

HISTORY

For at least 5000 years, as evidenced in the Edwin Smith Surgical Papyrus from Egypt, symptoms of incontinence, cystitis, prostatitis, and urethritis have been studied by examination of the urine. Because *Schistosoma haematobium* was common, primitive Egyptians wore various sheaths over the penis to prevent entry of parasites into the body. The urethral orifice was considered mystical; urine was curious and magical (31). The use of such sheaths has been more recently observed in primitive Amazon tribes.

In all primitive tribes and in mythical English literature there is a litany of folklore regarding urine. The conversion of consumed water and wine into urine was recognized, and most butchers recognized the kidneys as the source of the water traveling down through ureters and into the bladder. The Greeks described and clearly recognized glomerulonephritis with statements such as "Sometimes blood bursts from the kidneys suddenly in large quantity and flows for many days. None, however, die from the hemorrhage itself, which usually stops . . ." (31). The related description of chronic nephritis noted that, when blood passed in the urine, it was often associated with headache, epileptic convulsions, dropsy, and paralysis.

In the thirteenth century, Actuarius of Constantinople published his book, *De Urinis*, in which he described urine color typical of paroxysmal hemoglobinuria. The sweet taste of urine in diabetes was known by the Ancients but was made a diagnostic criteria by the Englishman Willis in 1674 (38).

The art of looking at urine in a glass to determine whether it is clear or cloudy, bloody, yellow, or white began, at least, with Hippocrates. This process is known as uroscopy and ultimately led to the microscopic examination of urine after the microscope was invented in the seventeenth century.

Bright, at Guy's Hospital in London, correlated autopsy findings of scarred kidneys with the clinical picture of edema and proteinuria and in

2   Introduction

1827 described the disease now known as Bright's disease (33). These renal specimens are available for view in the museum at Guy's Hospital. Current diagnosis of these specimens indicates they represent a mixed group of patients who had not only glomerulonephritis but also pyelonephritis and hypertensive vascular disease. Prout, a colleague of Bright's, began routine testing of urine for volume, color, specific gravity, and pH, as well as protein testing by heat coagulation. In 1833 Bence–Jones discovered that urinary protein could be coagulated by heat and that with further heating the coagulum would later redissolve (33).

Tubular casts were observed in kidney tissue when specimens from Guy's Hospital were studied under the newer nineteenth century microscopes, providing early insight into the place of origin of casts and modern recognition of the multiple types of kidney disease (33).

ROUTINE URINALYSIS AND ITS SIGNIFICANCE

The kidney is vital to life and exists as the regulator of internal biochemistry in blood and body fluids. Its processes of first filtering the blood through the glomerulus, regulating the size of protein molecules which may enter the tubules through filtration, and passing this filtrate through the renal tubules where processes of absorption and secretion modify the composition, significantly influence the pH, P_{CO_2}, and bicarbonate of the blood and of the final excretion product. Within the renal tubules, processes of reabsorption and secretion occur, resulting in modification of the filtrate. The final product excreted from the tubules is much different in composition from the initial filtrate and much reduced in volume.

The kidney is structured to excrete metabolic wastes while conserving body water, achieving this by the production of hypertonic urine. It is the principal site for excretion of end products of nitrogen metabolism.

The excreted urine contains urochromes, may contain drugs ingested, and may or may not reflect internal disease of the kidneys or body as a whole. However, certain excretion products, such as Bence–Jones proteins, specifically reflect the erroneous synthesis of gamma globulins in plasma cells which are far removed from the kidney.

Normally, the total amount of dissolved constituents excreted in 24 hours is about 60 g, which is proportioned as follows (53):

Organic (35 g)
1. Urea
2. Uric acid
3. Creatinine

Inorganic (25 g)
1. Ammonia
2. Chlorides
3. Sulphates
4. Phosphates
} Associated with hydrogen, sodium, potassium, magnesium, calcium, etc.

In the normal adult, blood passes through the kidney (Fig. 1–1) at a rate of about 1.2 liters/min, of which 720 ml is plasma; about one-fifth of the plasma is filtered through the glomeruli. The ultrafiltrate contains virtually all of the nonprotein components of plasma. The pH and osmolality of the filtrate are the same as those of plasma. To maintain homeostasis, this filtrate is modified by several distinct mechanisms as it passes down the tubule into the urinary bladder. Glucose, amino acids, proteins, sodium, potassium, phosphates, uric acid, chlorides, and bicarbonate are variably reabsorbed from the proximal tubule. Secretion of uric acid, potassium, hydrogen ion, and other substances such as glucuronides and penicillins is accomplished along the renal tubule or nephron unit. These processes are variably linked to negative feedback mechanisms that respond to aldosterone, P_{CO_2}, cellular level of potassium, or other as yet unidentified substances (66).

The next major site of reabsorption is in the thick, ascending limb of the loop of Henle. Here chloride is actively reabsorbed, with sodium passively following. Calcium and magnesium are also reabsorbed in this section of the nephron.

Fig. 1–1. Normal human kidneys, ureters, and their attachment to the urinary bladder.

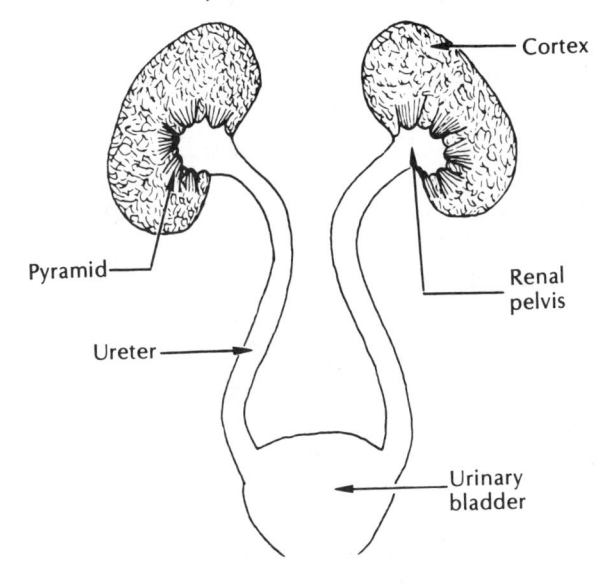

About 90% of the fluid is reabsorbed by the time the ultrafiltrate reaches the distal tubule whether the subject is in a state of hydration or dehydration. In the distal tubule and collecting duct more water is reabsorbed under the regulatory influence of antidiuretic hormone (ADH) which maintains water homeostasis. At this distal site under the influence of aldosterone, both acidification of the urine and potassium secretion occur, along with the final regulation of substances that were not reabsorbed in the proximal tubule.

In general, the composition of the urine reflects the status of hydration, the dietary intake, and the basal metabolic production of many of the substances mentioned. To assess abnormality, one must have knowledge of 1) potassium intake or potassium balance, 2) sodium intake or sodium balance, 3) fluid intake in assessing impairment of renal concentrating ability, and 4) the previous exercise or body temperature of the patient in assessing protein excretion in the urine (66).

Urea constitutes about half (20–35 g) of the total dissolved solids in 24 hours. The chlorides, practically all in the form of sodium chloride, make up about half (4–8 g) of the inorganic substances in 24 hours (Table 1–1).

TABLE 1-1. URINARY CONSTITUENTS (24 HR) OF THE AVERAGE ADULT ON AN AVERAGE DIET

Constituent	Blood level (mg/100 ml)	Quantity in urine (g)	Quantity filtered* (g)	Amount reabsorbed (g)	(%)
Amino acid N	10 ± 5	0.1–0.2	18.0	17.85	99.1
Ammonia N	0.024 ± 0.020	0.3–1.2	0.045	0†	—
Bicarbonate	27 ± 5 mM	2.0–3.0 mM	4,860 mM	4,858.0 mM	99.9
Calcium	10 ± 1	0.1–0.3	18.0	17.8	98.8
Chloride	365 ± 10	4.0–8.0	657.0	651.0	99.0
Creatinine	1.0 ± 0.5	1.2–1.8	1.8	0†	—
Glucose (fasting state)	85 ± 20	0	180.0	180.0	100.0
Magnesium	1.75 ± 0.25	0.1–0.2	3.15	3.0	95.0
Phosphate	3.5 ± 0.5	0.5–1.5	6.3	5.3	84.0
Potassium	19 ± 3	2.5–3.0	36.0	33.5	93.5
Sodium	325 ± 15	2.0–5.0	585.0	582.0	99.6
Sulfate (as S)	1.5 ± 0.3	0.5–1.0	2.7	2.0	74.0
Urea	27 ± 7	20.0–35.0	48.6	24.3	50.0‡
Uric acid	3 ± 1	0.4–1.0	5.4	4.7	87.0

*If the glomerular filtration rate is 130 ml/min.
†Tubular excretion, rather than reabsorption, occurs.
‡Varies with the rate of urine flow (40–60%).

(Baird EE: Ch 1, Vol 4. In Race GJ (ed): Laboratory Medicine. Hagerstown, Harper & Row, 1978)

Increased concentrations of certain substances appear in the urine in pathologic conditions, the most important of these being proteins, sugars, ketone bodies, bile (bilirubin), porphyrins, porphobilinogen, urobilinogen, and hemoglobin. In addition, urine contains hormones in varying concentrations and various microscopic structures such as crystals, casts, cells, bacteria, etc.

The average daily output of urine is normally 750–2000 ml; amounts greater or less than this range are usually considered pathologic. Normally, three to four times more urine is excreted during the day (8:00 A.M. to 8:00 P.M.) than during the night (8:00 P.M. to 8:00 A.M.). It is evident therefore that the time of collection is important and that no quantitative test can be of any value unless the urine sample has been collected during a known interval of time.

For most clinical purposes, a random voided specimen is adequate for qualitative examination. The first urine voided in the morning is usually the most suitable since this specimen is likely to have the most uniform volume and concentration.

The urine must be examined while fresh. Decomposition sets in rapidly, especially at warm temperatures, and interferes with all estimations.

PURPOSE OF URINALYSIS

Most laboratory procedures are performed to verify or disprove a diagnostic hypothesis previously gained by evaluation of a patient's history and physical findings (2). Mass screening has been justified only when the procedure is used in the detection of a disease entity that has one or more of the following characteristics: 1) occurs with a relatively high incidence in the general population; 2) has a silent symptomatology during the early stages or has such protean manifestations as to preclude clinical recognition; 3) characteristically produces sequelae that are of serious consequences; or 4) is used in screening for drugs. There are only four laboratory procedures that readily meet these requirements: a blood examination for evidence of either anemia or infection; a blood test for detecting evidence suggestive of syphilis; a test performed on newborns for phenylketonuria; and a routine urinalysis for evidences of local renal pathology, generalized metabolic disturbances, or drugs.

The routine urinalysis is a valuable screening procedure whose primary aims are threefold: 1) to check grossly for the possible existence of diabetes mellitus; 2) to check roughly for an acid–base, fluid, or electrolyte imbalance; and 3) to check for the presence or absence of an inflammatory process in the genitourinary system. Occasionally some inferential information on one function of the renal tubular or nephron unit is derived from the routine urinalysis through the determination of specific gravity.

All too frequently, these potential values inherent in the screening urinalysis are overshadowed by its failure to measure more of the kidney's true functional capacity. The value lies in its being a relatively inexpensive and easy to perform procedure that yields valuable diagnostic information that might not otherwise be ascertained. For example, diabetes mellitus, which occurred in approximately 10 million people in the United States in 1977, would remain unrecognized in many instances until the crisis of diabetic coma supervened if screening urinalysis were not utilized for its detection (65).

The various types of nephritides frequently fail to demonstrate localizing signs and may manifest with only such vague constitutional symptoms as general malaise and fever. This lack of localizing symptoms is especially common in children, and routine urinalysis frequently indicates that the cause of the illness is located in the urinary tract.

It is suggested that the routine urinalysis include the following observations:

1. Physical characteristics
   a. Specific gravity
   b. Color, only if abnormal
   c. Transparency
   d. Odor
2. Chemical characteristics
   a. Glucose
   b. Acetone
   c. Protein
   d. Bile pigments
3. Microscopic examination of the sediment (concentrated 20:1) showing normal or increased numbers of
   a. Leukocytes (pus cells) per high-powered field (HPF)
   b. Erythrocytes per HPF
   c. Casts per low-powered field (LPF), indicating type
   d. Bacteria
   e. Crystals per LPF

Each of these determinations affords useful information to the clinician for either detecting or excluding the possibility of diabetes mellitus, ketosis, or inflammation within the genitourinary tract.

2 Specimen Collection and Preservation

The technique used to collect the urine sample and the handling of the specimen before urinalysis is of critical importance in interpretation of the laboratory findings.

COLLECTION METHODS

Several different methods can be used to collect the specimen.

VOIDED SAMPLE

The entire voided sample is collected. This is the usual type of collection in a routine screening procedure. However, utilization of this technique in collecting samples from females results in specimens which are impossible to interpret microscopically because the collected urine represents a mixture of urine and vaginal fluids.

THREE-GLASS URINE

The act of voiding is divided into three segments: 1) the first glass contains the initial 10–30 cc; 2) the second glass holds the midportion of the voided sample—usually 30–150 cc; and 3) the third portion is that voided just at the termination of urination—usually 15–30 cc. These samples need to be carefully marked and treated separately. The three-glass urine collection, used primarily for the male, is designed to permit sampling from different levels of the urinary tract. The first glass contains a urethral sample; the second glass, a bladder sample; and the third glass, a contribution of the prostatic urethra. (As micturition is completed, the prostatic tissues contract resulting in additional secretions to the urine.)

MIDSTREAM URINE

Midstream urine is the sample of urine collected from the bladder, similar to that contained in the second glass of urine in the three-glass technique. The technique of collection is of critical importance. In the male, a midstream specimen is best collected in the standing position. Prior to collection, the glans penis is wiped with a swab moistened with an antiseptic agent. Urination is then begun, and a cup is thrust into the midportion of the urinary stream and withdrawn before urination is terminated. In the female, the labia need to be spread and held apart. The urethral orifice is wiped with a swab moistened with an antiseptic agent with a motion in a posterior direction, toward the anus. This preparation is often facilitated by the patient's sitting backwards on the toilet seat. After urination has commenced, the sample is collected by thrusting a cup into the urine stream.

CATHETER SPECIMEN("IN-AND-OUT" BLADDER CATHETERIZATION)

On occasion, especially in the female, a catheter is used to obtain a urine sample not contaminated with vaginal contents. Also, in either sex, catheterization may be required because of difficulty in passing urine. A urine sample may be submitted after such a procedure. In each instance, the sample is collected from the open end of the catheter.

The collection of urine from an indwelling bladder catheter must be carefully obtained for proper interpretation. The catheter and drainage system is not disconnected. A sterile syringe with a 1-in., 25-gauge needle is used to puncture the catheter itself or a special area on the drainage tubing adjacent to its connection with the catheter after sterile cleansing of the site with an iodine type antiseptic, and a sample is aspirated.

URETEROILEOSTOMY SAMPLE

On occasion the ureters are surgically removed from the bladder and reimplanted into an isolated loop of ileum. The urine exists from a stoma on the anterior abdominal wall. A reliable sample can only be collected by passing a sterile catheter through the stoma into the ileal segment and aspirating the sample. Samples collected from the ileostomy bag are invariably so heavily contaminated with bacteria as to produce severe interpretive problems.

URETERAL SAMPLE

During the procedure of retrograde ureteral catheterization, samples are occasionally collected from each ureter. Careful labeling, distinguishing one side from the other, is mandatory. These samples are usually submitted for culture as well as urinalysis.

SUPRAPUBIC ASPIRATION OF THE BLADDER

As a substitute for in-and-out catheterization of the bladder, a sample can be obtained by inserting a 21-gauge spinal needle into the distended bladder. The aspirated sample is especially useful when looking for pyuria and bacteria in the female, as vaginal contamination of voided urine is a problem.

HANDLING THE SPECIMEN

Prompt delivery of the collected specimen to the laboratory and rapid analysis are essential for a meaningful interpretation. Urine is subject to rapid decomposition at room temperature, i.e., casts may dissolve, cells disintegrate, urea may be converted into ammonia by bacterial action, and bacteria may proliferate. Specimens should be brought to the laboratory within 30 min of collection. Should unavoidable delay occur, the specimen may be refrigerated; however, this delay should not exceed 2 hours. Once the sample has arrived, no delay should occur before analysis is performed.

Samples which do not meet the criteria for collection or delivery should be identified and appropriately marked as possibly unacceptable samples. However, an analysis should proceed. Often the urine has been collected at a critical time or during a procedure which cannot be repeated. Discarding such a sample would not be in the best interest of the patient. However, the clinician should be advised of the criteria violated so that the results of analysis can be properly interpreted.

SPECIMEN PRESERVATION

Preservation of the specimen is necessary because the collecting technique is not sterile and usually results in a heavy bacterial growth after several hours unless the sample is refrigerated. These organisms may utilize glucose as a source of energy and change a positive test for glycosuria into a negative one; if the bacterial flora is great enough, the bacterial proteins may give a false-positive test for proteinuria. Many of the bacteria are urea splitters. Their formation of ammonia from the urea makes the specimen alkaline, a pH at which casts promptly dissolve. Thus, for several reasons, the urinalysis should be made promptly or steps to preserve the specimen should be taken.

There are several methods of preservation, all of which are bacteriostatic in principle and most of which interfere in one way or another in the urinalysis procedure. The choice of the preservative, as well as the decision on whether one should be used at all, should reside with the laboratory personnel. (This is not the case with a 24-hour specimen when part of the sample remains on the ward for many hours). The examiner knows whether there will be an appreciable delay in making the analysis and knows which interference may be expected from which preservative.

The following methods of preserving a specimen of urine are listed in the order of descending desirability:

1. Refrigeration. This is the most desirable method as it creates no distortion of formed elements and interferes only with the test for specific gravity. The lack of refrigerating facilities usually limits this method of preservation to a few specimens.
2. Toluene. A few milliliters of toluene provide good bacteriostasis and do not interfere with any of the routine chemical determinations. However, toluene floats on the surface of the specimen, creating a slight nuisance for the examiner.
3. Formalin. About one drop/ounce of urine not only serves to inhibit bacterial growth but also preserves casts and cellular elements. Unfortunately, formalin's aldehyde radical also reduces the occasionally used Benedict's solution and causes a false-positive test for sugar; in addition, formalin interferes with such nonroutine procedures as Obermayer's test for indican.
4. Benzoate–Urotropin (methanamine) tablet. The Association of Life Insurance Directors has endorsed the preservation of urine for mailing by using one tablet of the following composition for each ounce of urine:

Monopotassium phosphate	100 mg
Benzoic acid	65 mg
Sodium benzoate	50 mg
Urotropin (methanamine)	50 mg
Sodium bicarbonate	10 mg
Red mercuric oxide	1 mg

5. Boric acid. A little more than 5 mg/ml urine is needed before any appreciable bacteriostatic influence is noted. At this concentration it may cause troublesome precipitates.
6. Chloroform. Although this reagent has been advocated for use as a preservative, it is quite inadequate except for aldosterone collection. It causes changes in the characteristics of the cellular sediment.
7. Vacuum drying or freezing. Leach (37) reported the following:

In preparation for the conduct of biochemical experiments in the Skylab Orbital Workshop, a study was performed on the stability of various chemical constituents in urine in two different techniques for preservation and storage. Urine samples were either vacuum dried or frozen and maintained in storage at $-20°$ for periods of up to 10 weeks. The urinary constituents studied included aldosterone, antidiuretic hormone, epinephrine, norepinephrine, urea, nitrogen, creatinine, hydroxyproline, 17-hydroxycorticosteroids, calcium, sodium, potassium, chloride, magnesium, and phosphate. Some degradation of urinary compounds was observed after both treatments. The rate and variability of destruction following the vacuum drying treatment, however, was greater than for freezing. It was concluded that only the freezing treatment could be used to preserve with predictable loss the urinary samples which would be returned to earth following the conclusion of each Skylab flight.

Cognizance should be taken of the fact that, besides the deterioration due to urine aging, there are various materials that may contaminate routinely collected specimens and vitiate the results of some of the procedures, e.g., contamination of unvoided urine caused by medications, contamination from the genitals during voiding, or contamination of voided urine caused by a chemically unclean container. Care must be taken to avoid such contaminations by using chemically clean containers and avoiding examination of a specimen obtained during the menses. The drug contaminations usually cannot be avoided, but allowances should be made for their influence upon the procedures.

PART II TESTING PROCEDURES

3 Physical Characteristics

COLOR

Urine may range from a deep amber color through varying tints of yellow to colorless, depending upon the concentration of urochrome, an endogenously formed, yellow brown pigment (20,21,43). The quantity of pigment produced and excreted is quite uniform during each hour of the day and does not vary with age, sex, diet, etc., although the quantity formed does bear a relationship to the individual's muscle mass. In accelerated rates of metabolism, such as with hyperpyrexia, there may be some acceleration of urochrome excretion. This constancy of the pigment excretion rate means that the intensity of color imparted to the urine depends exclusively upon the volume of urine formed per unit of time. For example, the small volume of night urine (about 20 ml/hour) is heavily colored because the 20 ml contain as much pigment as the 150 ml or more of urine that would be formed in 1 hour following a large fluid intake during the day.

One function of the kidney is to remove from the blood all soluble foreign substances and worthless metabolites. Occasionally these are colored substances, and in rare instances the color of the urine may be diagnostically suggestive. The most frequent cause of an abnormal urine color is medication, but seldom does the clinician need to rely upon the color of the urine to indicate medications administered. However, since an abnormal color may have significance, it is recommended that the reporting of abnormal colors be a part of a screening urinalysis. Some of the common causes for an abnormal color of the urine are given in Table 3-1. Kilduffe (35) may be consulted for a more complete list.

TABLE 3-1. ABNORMAL URINE COLORS

Color	Caused by drug or food	Caused by disease or condition
Red	Beets, phenolphthalein, (alkaline), eosin, Pyridium, sulfomethanes, selenium, Mercurochrome (instilled), aminophenazone	Porphyrinuria, hematuria (gross) hemoglobinuria, increased urobilinogen production
Brown or red brown	Rhubarb, senna, cascara, Argyrol (instilled)	Gross hematuria (smoky), hemolysis, increased myoglobin production, old blood, melanin (turns black on oxidation)
Pale green, green, or blue green	Phenyl salicylate, methylene blue, phenol, bromoforium, diagnex blue, indigo carmine	Bilirubinurias, (biliverdin), occasionally in diabetes mellitus
Black or gray	Phenyl salicylate (when excessive in amount)	Melanosis, alkaptonuria, old blood
Amber or orange or excessive yellow	Azogantrisin or Pyridium; multivitamins, especially thiamine HCl	Urobilinogen, bilirubin, normal urochromes
White or pink cloudy	Only under turbidity	Chyluria, pyuria

(Modified from Baird EE: Ch 1, Vol 4. In Race GJ (ed): Laboratory Medicine. Hagerstown, Harper & Row, 1978)

CLARITY

Urine is generally clear. Cloudiness in the urine usually is due to amorphous phosphates, which are white sediments in alkaline urine that disappear when acid is added. Amorphous phosphate precipitates are very common and often represent no clinical importance, especially when the urine is relatively alkaline (Table 3-1).

Amorphous urates are less common, and the urine takes on a white or pink, cloudy, "brick dust" appearance which will disappear upon heating.

Pus may look like amorphous phosphates, but turbidity increases when acid is added to the urine. A gelatin is formed in the presence of heavy pus when NaOH is added (Donné test).

A bloody, reddish brown or smoky colored urine gives the gross impression that there is hematuria, hemoglobinuria, or myoglobinuria; but this must be confirmed microscopically and chemically.

Bacteria can produce cloudiness, especially in old urine which has been allowed to stand at room temperature.

ODOR

Usually the odor of urine is associated with its deterioration and is of little significance. The odor of urine from growth of bacteria may be pungent, typical of gram-negative bacteria or ammonia. Ammonia produced by bacterial splitting of urea is common. However, in ketonuria, acetone or diacetic acids may give a sweet or fruity smell. A very foul-smelling urine is usually a sign of infection with gross contamination by pus. The excretion of urine which smells like maple syrup indicates a congenital metabolic defect.

FOAM

Urine usually is not foamy, but yellow foam will increase following excretion of bilirubin. Surface tension is altered and any agitation produces foam. This observation is the basis for one of the tests for bilirubinuria.

High protein concentration in urine will alter surface tension and also produce foam.

4 Specific Gravity and Osmolality

One of the very important functions of the kidney is to vary the amount of water removed from the urine as it passes through the tubular system of the kidney. This process is accomplished by the tubular structures of the kidney. A hormone elaborated from the hypothalamic-posterior pituitary portion of the brain, the antidiuretic hormone (ADH), plays a critical role in controlling this process.

The initially formed urine (glomerular filtrate) contains the same amount of water as plasma. A urine more dilute than plasma is formed when chemical substances are removed from the glomerular filtrate. The net removal of water from the glomerular filtrate results in a fluid more concentrated than plasma.

SPECIFIC GRAVITY

Specific gravity is the measure of the density of a solution. Water is used as the point of reference and is assigned a specific gravity of 1.000. The addition of solute to water increases its specific gravity. Plasma has a specific gravity of 1.010. A urine with a specific gravity of less than 1.010 is dilute in comparison to plasma; the elaboration of such a urine is referred to as **hyposthenuria**. The elaboration of a urine with a specific gravity the same as plasma, *i.e.*, 1.010, is referred to as **isosthenuria**. The elaboration of a urine with a specific gravity greater than 1.010 is more concentrated than plasma and is referred to as **hyperosthenuria**. The urine specific gravity from a normal subject varies with the need of the individual to conserve or excrete water and hence varies 1.003–1.040. Values for urine are never below 1.003. On occasion, a specific gravity greater than 1.040 is observed if the urine contains radiographic contrast agents, dextrans, or an extraordinary amount of glucose.

The specific gravity varies with the fluid intake of the normal individual (Table 4–1). Abnormal results occur when the urine is inappropriately dilute or concentrated to the body's needs. For example, the elaboration of a dilute urine at a time when the individual is dehydrated would suggest either the absence of ADH, an insensitivity to its action, or the effect of a drug. Similarly, if the individual has excess body fluids, the elaboration of a concentrated urine in the absence of glucose, protein, or exogenously administered compounds of high density such as x-ray agents or dextrans may also suggest an abnormal response of the kidney.

TABLE 4-1. CHANGES IN URINARY CHARACTERISTICS WHEN THE KIDNEY CANNOT PERFORM OSMOTIC WORK

Parameter	Normal	Impaired osmotic function
Volume (ml)		
Day	950 ± 200	1100 ± 300
Night	250 ± 100	700 ± 200
Total (24 hours)	1200 ± 300	1800 ± 300
Day/night ratio	4:1	2:1 or 1:1
Nocturia	—	+++
Specific gravity		
Pooled day	1.014 ± 0.003	1.010 ± 0.002
Pooled night	1.030 ± 0.005	1.010 ± 0.002
Pooled 24 hour	1.018 ± 0.003	1.010 ± 0.002
Lowest single specimen	1.003 ± 0.002	1.010 ± 0.002
Highest single specimen	1.035 ± 0.003	1.010 ± 0.002

(Baird EE: Ch 1, Vol 4. In Race GJ (ed): Laboratory Medicine. Hagerstown, Harper & Row, 1978)

The measurement of specific gravity (but not osmolality) is affected by the presence of molecules of high density dissolved in the urine. These may be endogenously produced, that is, glucose or protein, or may be exogenously administered and appear in the urine, *i.e.*, x-ray contrast agents or dextran. A urine protein concentration of 1 g/dl generally elevates the specific gravity by 1.003. A urine glucose concentration of 1 g/dl raises the specific gravity by 1.004. In addition, variations of temperature may affect the specific gravity unless internally corrected by the specific gravity method.

METHODS OF TESTING SPECIFIC GRAVITY
HYDROMETER (URINOMETER)

A weighted float is placed in a column of still urine. The level to which the float sinks is a measure of the specific gravity. The float is actually displacing a certain weight of urine which represents specific gravity. This can be measured by reading a calibration on the side of the float. Care should be taken to assure that there is a clear meniscus, that there are no bubbles or foam on the surface, that the depth of the column of the urine is adequate, and that the float does not touch the sides of the vessel. The usual urinometer is not temperature corrected, although it can be, and the urine should be at 20°C. For each 3° decrement below 20°C, a correction factor of 0.001 should be subtracted.

The urinometer should be so calibrated that distilled water at 20°C reads exactly 1.000. A graduated or ungraduated cylinder used to contain the urine should be of sufficient diameter to prevent the urinometer's adherence to the sides when it is twirled with the fingers. One should make the reading at the point where the bottom of the meniscus contacts the urinometer.

REFRACTOMETER

The refractometer measures the density of a solution by the angle that transmitted light is affected by the solution's density. The refractometer is temperature compensated.

A few drops of urine are placed in the sample chamber, and the reading is immediately determined. This provides a rapid, accurate measurement of specific gravity.

SEMIAUTOMATED DEVICE

A semiautomated device for measuring specific gravity has been devised with electrical weighing of a float suspended in the urine sample.

OSMOLALITY

The measurement of osmolality is a more meaningful parameter in the assessment of concentration and dilution functions of the kidney. This measurement is a function of the number of dissolved particles in a solution. It is not affected by the size of the particle as is the specific gravity, and it can be more accurately measured. In dilute solutions, the milliosmole concentration is nearly the same as the millimole concentration. However, the preparation of any standard solution should take into consideration the osmotic coefficient.

The osmolality of plasma is 285–290 mOsm/kg water (hereafter referred to as mOsm). A urine with an osmolality of less than plasma is regarded as dilute. The lowest achievable osmolality in urine is 50 mOsm. A urine with an osmolality greater than plasma is considered concentrated. The highest achievable osmolality of human urine is about 1200 mOsm.

The osmolality of the urine may be appropriate to requirements of the individual. The capability of modern instruments to measure more precisely and reproducibly the osmolality has proved measurement to be the best indicator of subtle abnormalities of the concentrating or diluting capacity of the kidneys. The osmolality of the urine is not affected by the presence of high density compounds in the urine (such as glucose, protein, dextrans, and radiographic contrast material). Further information may be gathered if the plasma and urine are obtained simultaneously and a direct comparison is made between the two.

The osmolality is determined by the depression of the freezing point or by the measurement of the dew point. The former method, available for several years, is rather nicely automated so that the specimen is thrust into a chilling well; the steps of chilling, seating, and temperature measurement are done automatically. With standard equipment, using freezing point depression to determine osmolality in microvolumes is often not as accurate unless microosmometers are used. The dew point type osmometer utilizes a 50-μl sample for analysis. While this new method may replace the freezing point depression technique, the latter method and equipment have stood the test of time.

5 Microscopic Examination

The technique for the examination of urine under the microscope has changed little over the years, and this visual microscopic examination is no less important in its significance or usefulness now than it was at its inception. Careful interpretation of the findings observed in examination of the urine sediment can provide rather accurate localizing information of pathologic processes in the urinary tract or, on occasion, point to a specific diagnosis or clinical problem. Therefore the urine sediment should be examined with care and with recognition of its significance (Col. Fig. 5-1).

METHOD

Proper care begins with the method of collection, *i.e.*, midstream, three-glass, catheterization, suprapubic aspiration, etc., and is followed by prompt delivery to the laboratory and rapid processing (see Collection Methods, Ch. 2).

Place about 10 ml of urine in a clinical test tube and centrifuge for 3-5 min at about 2000 RPM. Decant the supernatant by rapid inversion of the tube, usually leaving about 0.5 ml urine sediment behind. Take one drop of the well-mixed sediment from the tip of the tube and transfer to a clean slide. A coverslip should be used. Cut down the transmitted light on the microscope by closing the iris and lowering the stage. The urine should be scanned under low power with the edge of the coverslip serving as a guide. The entire perimeter of the coverslip should be observed. This scanning procedure can be interrupted for higher power observations of an interesting or infrequent finding but then should be continued. As this is being done, a general estimate of elements noted on low-power scan can be recorded, *i.e.*, epithelial cells, mucus, crystals (type), sperm, yeast, parasites, etc. The urine sample should then be subjected to high-power inspection. Earlier in the scanning procedure specific areas of interest had been examined and noted (such as type of casts or crystals). Now the specific examination of the number of white and red cells per HPF should be estimated. In order to provide a reasonably accurate estimate, a field in each corner of the coverslip and the central areas should be examined.

FINDINGS AND INTERPRETATIONS

LEUKOCYTES

A few leukocytes are present in normal urine but should not exceed three to four per HPF in the centrifuged specimen. Unstained leukocytes in a fluid medium present a vastly different appearance than they do in either a histologic section or stained blood film. They appear smaller ($10-12\mu$), are more spherical in a fluid environment, and can be identified quite easily by their characteristic granularity or the lobulations of the nucleus that often exist. A few drops of acetic acid added to the urine sediment enhances the identifying granularity, but the acid is generally not needed. On occasion, the leukocytes may have been produced in sufficient numbers to group together. This finding should be reported as clumps of white blood cells (WBCs).

It must be remembered that leukocytes possess ameboid characteristics; cells exhibiting such activity, while infrequently seen, should not *per se* suggest parasitism. Also, it should be recalled that in an environment such as urine, all cells undergo various osmotically imposed changes that eventually produce death and dissolution. Some of the earlier degenerating changes occurring in leukocytes include the disappearance of the nucleus and the appearance of refractile fatty materials called myelin droplets.

An increase in leukocytes in the urine is associated with an inflammatory process any place in or adjacent to the urinary tract. Under the influence of chemotaxis, leukocytes are attracted to any area of inflammation and, with their ameboid properties, penetrate all areas adjacent to the inflammatory site. Sometimes pyuria is seen in such conditions as appendicitis, salpingitis, and pancreatitis. Those cells that invade the lumen of the urinary tract may do so at any place between the glomerulus of the kidney and the meatus of the urethra. They are then washed away by the flow of the urine and voided with it.

Comment should be made regarding the apparent significance of "glitter" cells in the urinary sediment. These cells are leukocytes that have become swollen and enlarged in the hypotonic urine. The cytoplasmic granules of such swollen cells exhibit brownian movement and have the appearance of glittering. Earlier authors postulated that these cells were diagnostic of pyelonephritis, but it is now understood that they occur in a great variety of conditions if cells are exposed to a hypotonic medium. It has been demonstrated that desquamated vaginal epithelial cells and even *Trichomonas vaginalis* organisms may exhibit this glitter phenomenon when devitalized and subjected for a prolonged period of time to the osmotic effect of a hypotonic environment; consequently, it seems very doubtful that these cells possess any special diagnostic value.

Staining of the leukocytes with Wright's stain may on occasion be helpful, especially if eosinophiluria is considered a possibility. To facilitate this examination, the urine sediment should be mixed with 0.5 cc of a plasma solution. The source of protein is unimportant and may consist of 5% bovine serum albumin. The urine sediment, protein mixture is smeared on a clean glass slide and allowed to dry. The dried sediment should then be stained with Wright's stain by the usual method. Any eosinophils in the urine are of importance and should be reported. This finding suggests an allergic interstitial nephritis.

Leukocytes are macrophages in the urinary tract and can incorporate fat (the latter present in heavy proteinuria); as a result, these fat-filled cells become very prominent, especially when viewed with polarized light. These fat-filled inclusions are brilliantly refractile and have a Maltese cross appearance.

ERYTHROCYTES

Normal urine should never contain more than a rare red cell per HPF in the centrifuged sediment unless the red cells represent a contamination (as from the vagina). When fresh, red cells have a normal appearance and are biconcave disks of uniform size; however, they may be swollen in dilute urine or crenated in concentrated urine. When they have been in the urine any considerable time, their hemoglobin may have dissolved; they may appear as faint, colorless circles and are more difficult to see. An estimated number of cells per HPF is recorded.

The identifying characteristics of erythrocytes are not quite as distinctive as those of leukocytes. Erythrocytes, after settling out in a liquid medium, appear in the microscopic field as rather uniformly round with rather faintly yellow bodies and a completely homogeneous structure. Occasionally, through osmotic action, red blood cells found in the urine possess refractile areas which suggest to the unwary that the cells contain nuclei. Observations of several of these cells usually permit recognition of this artifact.

A more frequent error is the identification of yeast cells as erythrocytes. This occurs because yeast cells infrequently contaminate old urine and bear a superficial resemblance to red blood cells; however, their characteristics permit relatively easy differentiation (Table 5-1).

The causes for hematuria are multiple. Since red blood cells should rarely be observed in the urine of normal individuals, hematuria, whether it be gross or microscopic, demands follow-up evaluation for its cause. Unlike leukocytes, the red blood cells have no ameboid properties and consequently remain within the blood vessels. They appear in the urine only following vascular injury which allows their escape. The vascular injury producing hematuria may be altered capillary permeability of an inflammatory process with hemorrhage by diapedesis into the urine or may be by traumatic damage to the vessels adjacent to the lumen of the urinary transport system.

On occasion, hemoglobin is detected in the urine, but no red blood cells

Col. Fig. 5-1. Plate 1. Microscopic Examination. **A.** Hyaline cast. **B.** RBC cast. **C.** Tubular epithelial cast. **D.** Waxy cast. **E.** Granular cast. **F.** Epithelial cells. **G.** WBC cast. **H.** Oval fat body. **I.** *Candida albicans* budding and RBCs. **J.** Triple phosphate crystals. **K.** Epithelial cells.

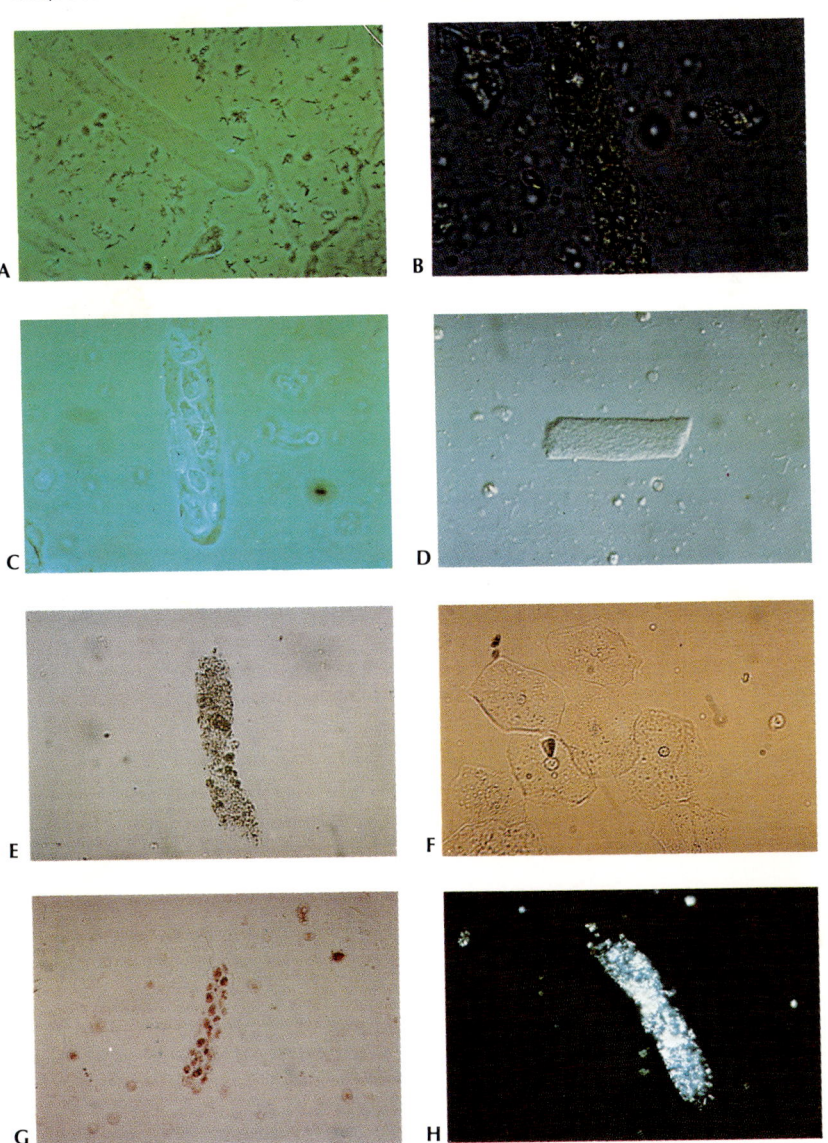

(Fig. 5-1. continued) **L.** Cystine crystals. **M.** RBCs and WBCs. **N.** Uric acid crystals. **O.** Magnesium phosphate. **P.** Uric acid cast (polarized). (Courtesy of Roche Laboratories, Division of Hoffman–LaRoche, Inc., Nutley, New Jersey).

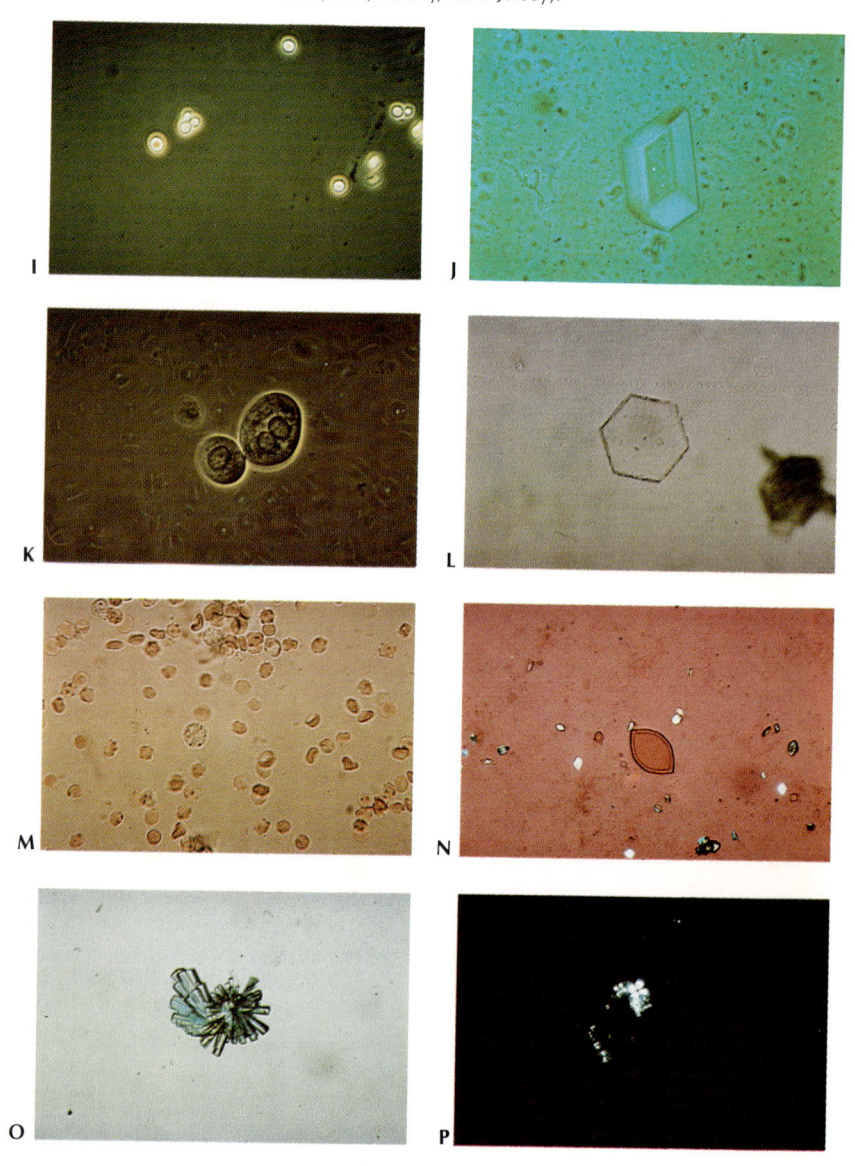

TABLE 5-1. DIFFERENTIATING CHARACTERISTICS BETWEEN ERYTHROCYTES AND YEAST CELLS

Parameter	Red cell	Yeast cell
Size (diameter)	Uniform, 6–7 μ	Variable (young buds), 3–5 μ
Shape	Round	Oval
Cell texture	Clear, hyalinelike; sharp cell membrane	Not hyaline, finely granular; cell membrane indistinct
	Faint yellow	White green
Budding	Never observed	Usually observed

(Baird EE: Ch 1, Vol 4. In Race GJ (ed): Laboratory Medicine. Hagerstown, Harper & Row, 1978)

are seen in the sediment. This observation may be of singular importance, for it strongly suggests that the pigment appearing in the urine (which may be hemoglobin or myoglobin) is originating from filtration of these products in the blood.

It should be noted that hematuria frequently is found in casually voided urine from adult females and is a result of residual menstrual flow or other forms of gynecologic bleeding.

EPITHELIAL CELLS

A distinguishing feature of the epithelial cell is a prominent nucleus in a clear cytoplasm. The ratio of cytoplasm to nucleus is variable. Epithelial cells may have such a large cytoplasm that they appear as "fried eggs." The cytoplasm of these cells may be so thin that the cells may be folded on themselves even in the thin film of urine sediment under a coverslip. On very rare occasions, the epithelial cells may have very distorted or irregular nuclei or may be undergoing mitosis. In such instances, these findings may suggest a malignant process of the cells lining the urinary tract.

BACTERIA, FUNGI, PARASITES

In a properly collected and processed specimen, the finding of bacteria may be of considerable importance. The process of centrifugation concentrates the bacteria and makes numerical quantification difficult. If bacteria are seen in the centrifuged specimens but not in the unspun urine sample, it suggests that less than 10,000 bacteria/ml are present. On the other hand, finding bacteria in an unspun sample of urine suggests that greater than 100,000 bacteria/ml are present.

Identification of the bacterial morphology can be obtained by a Gram stain of the sediment performed in the microbiology laboratory. *Mycobacterium tuberculosis* can be identified in the concentrated urine sediment by the use of acid-fast stains. This examination is best done in the microbiology laboratory.

Candida albicans is the most common fungus to appear in the urine. Differentiation of these organisms from red cells is important (Table 5–1). These fungi may appear as budding yeast or exhibit the formation of mycelia. The budding yeast appearance indicates that the fungi are coexisting with the host, while the mycelialike appearance is felt to reflect tissue invasion by the fungus. Other fungi such as *Cryptococcus*, *histoplasma* etc., on very rare occasions may be present in the urinary tract.

Several parasites may be found in the urine. The site of origin may be the urinary tract or, in the female, the vagina. In each instance, the finding is of importance. Less commonly seen forms should be confirmed by a trained parasitologist.

The parasite most often seen in urine is the flagellate *Trichomonas vaginalis hominis*. The incidence of this type of parasitism is very high in women and may be the cause of an intense vaginitis. In males, the parasite causes an asymptomatic urethritis. The bobbing type of motion in the organism readily identifies it as a flagellate; because *Trichomonas vaginalis hominis* is the only flagellate appearing in urine, identification is rapid and simple.

Trematodes are rarely seen in the United States but represent a major health problem in certain areas of North and Central America and North Africa. The urine may contain the egg that is characteristic of *Schistosoma haematobium* (North Africa) or *Schistosoma mansoni* (Puerto Rico, Central America). Needless to say, identification of these parasites in the urine would be of great clinical importance and especially so in an area where they would be unexpected.

Even less commonly, the urine may reveal pinworm eggs or remnants of echinococcal infestation.

CRYSTALS

Urine is usually supersaturated with several different chemicals at any one time. The factors maintaining these chemicals in the supersaturated state are complex but in part include temperature and pH. After urine has been voided and allowed to stand, these factors, which have prevented crystal formation, are partially removed; crystal formation occurs. As a consequence, the formation of some crystals should be regarded as an artifact of the system of collection.

In an acid urine one may see:

1. Uric acid. These crystals may occur in many shapes, the most characteristic being diamonds, rosettes, and cubes. Recognition depends less on the shape of the crystals than on the color (yellow or reddish brown). The acid pH of the urine and the fact that the crystals are soluble in sodium hydroxide and insoluble in hydrochloric or acetic acid aid in identification. Almost all colored crystals found in an acid urine can safely be considered uric acid unless the shape is especially characteristic of a different chemical crystalline compound. These may be associated with increased urate production (as in the case of treated leukemia), gout of the excessive production type, generalized muscle necrosis, etc. While the finding of uric acid or urate crystals in the urine may not be specific for a disease state, there are instances when such a finding is of substantial importance.
2. Amorphous urates. These are fine, yellowish, dark granules which disappear when heated and are readily soluble in sodium hydroxide.
3. Calcium oxalate. These are colorless, glistening, octahedral crystals, usually appearing as small squares crossed by two intersecting lines, but they may take a number of other shapes. They are dissolved by concentrated hydrochloric acid and recrystallize upon the addition of ammonia. These crystals are the most commonly occurring ones in acid urine.

In alkaline urines one may see:
1. Triple phosphate. These are three-sided, prism-shaped crystals. They have no pathologic significance and usually indicate that the urine specimen has been standing for some time.
2. Calcium phosphate. These needlelike prisms are most commonly thin, irregular, granular plates and are of little importance. They are also often seen in neutral or acid urine.
3. Amorphous phosphates. These dark granules, forming in an alkaline pH and frequently clumped together, will dissolve upon the addition of acetic acid.
4. Calcium carbonate. These may be mingled with the phosphate deposits as amorphous granules or colorless spheres. They are soluble in acetic acid but differ from phosphates in that gas is formed when they dissolve.
5. Ammonia biurate. These crystals are opaque, yellow, and usually seen as spheres covered by coarse spines or spicules. Upon the addition of acetic acid, they dissolve and plates of uric acid appear.

Cystine crystals may be found in an acid urine and appear as colorless, highly refractile, rather thick, hexagonal plates with well-defined edges, single or superimposed to form regular clusters. Uric acid sometimes may have a form that mimics cystine crystals, and cystinuria must be excluded.

Cystine is soluble in hydrochloric acid and insoluble in acetic acid. These crystals are rarely seen and are associated with congenital disorders (see Screening for Disorders, Cystinuria, Ch. 15).

Uric acid and urate crystals are refracted by utilizing polarized light. This is especially helpful in their identification.

Xanthine crystals may appear in the urine of those patients who produce large amounts of purine or who have been given allopurinol. The appearance of xanthine crystals is similar to that of uric acid.

CASTS

Casts serve as an important finding in localizing pathologic processes of the kidney. While all casts do not imply renal disease, they all arise from the kidney. The process which leads to cast formation is unknown, but it is thought to reflect the accumulation of debris in the tubular lumen. This debris may be the result of precipitation of protein in the tubular lumen as water is reabsorbed, or it may reflect the shedding of tubular inflammatory cells or red blood cells in the lumen which become entrapped in their own debris or in a proteinaceous gel already forming. These casts are extruded from the tubular system by the hydrostatic pressure of the formed urine behind them. Once in the bladder urine, the casts undergo a process of degradation, especially in an alkaline urine.

During examination, casts are best seen near the edge of the coverslip. They are reported as numbers per LPF and have the following classifications:

1. Hyaline casts. Typically these are colorless, homogeneous, semitransparent, cylindrical structures with parallel sides and rounded ends. Hyaline casts can be either straight or curved and may extend in length across several fields, although they are generally much shorter. These are the least significant of all casts; however they are occasionally of some clinical importance. They are usually stained yellow when the urine contains much bile. Hyaline casts are best seen when the light transluminating the urine is dimmed.
2. Waxy casts. These are more opaque than the hyaline variety and are usually shorter and broader with irregular, broken ends which sometimes appear to be segmented. Waxy casts are usually gray but may be colorless or yellowish and have a refractile appearance. They occur in most cases of advanced nephritis and are regarded as unfavorable signs.
3. Granular casts. These are hyaline casts in which numerous granules are embedded. Granular casts are classified as either finely granular or coarsely granular. Finely granular casts are grayish or yellow and con-

tain many fine granules. Coarsely granular casts are darker brown and contain large granules. These granules may be the result of degenerated cells which were entrapped in cast formation.
4. White blood cell casts (WBC casts). These casts contain large numbers of WBCs, which originate in the kidney. WBC casts are seen in cases of renal parenchymal inflammation such as pyelonephritis, interstitial nephritis, etc.
5. Red blood cell casts (RBC casts). In most cases these are identifiable by their color, which is bright orange or reddish brown. RBC casts may be called hemoglobin casts and are seen in acute glomerulonephritis, systemic lupus erythematosus, and other glomerular disorders of the kidney.

Identification of casts is of special importance in locating the origin of blood appearing in the urine. RBC casts indicate the kidney as the source; therefore, it is very important to identify RBC casts properly and exclude those casts of uncertain etiology.

One also must be very careful to distinguish between RBC casts and the fortuitous collection of RBCs. Features which permit this distinction include the presence of significant amounts of mucus in the urine and the absence of a surrounding halo of hyaline as is usually the case with RBC casts and the variability of appearance when mucus and RBCs simulate RBC casts.

Bacterial Casts

Bacterial casts consist of bacteria incorporated into the protein matrix of the cast. Almost always, the presence of bacterial casts indicates severe pyelonephritis.

Fatty Casts

Fatty casts contain numerous fat droplets from epithelial cell degeneration or from the incorporation of fat filtered into the glomerulus with macrophages. These droplets become entrapped in the cast meshwork.

Pigmented Casts

Casts of a variety of types (hyaline, cellular, or waxy) may have brownish to yellowish tinge. This pigmentation may represent hemoglobin breakdown, myoglobin, or occasionally other pigments.

Structures Mistaken for Casts

Many structures may be mistaken for casts: mucous threads; masses of urates, phosphates, or minute crystals; oval fat bodies, etc. Mucous threads appear as long threads or as more ribbonlike than hyaline casts. Mucous threads have less well-defined edges, and their ends may taper to a point or may be split or curled. These should not be confused with urethral plugs which are macroscopic. Masses of urates, phosphates, or minute crystals or masses which accidentally take a cylindrical form, possibly due to molding within the renal tubules, may closely resemble granular casts. Gentle heating or adding appropriate solvents will distinguish them from casts. Oval fat bodies are elements of clinical significance and are usually encountered in the urine of patients with nephrotic syndrome. These fat bodies consist of fat molecules which, because of the "leaky" glomerular capillary membrane, have appeared in the urine and may be free floating or trapped in macrophages.

TELESCOPED SEDIMENT

Although it is a poor term, telescoped sediment is used to describe the findings in the urinary sediment of a coexisting and chronic nephritic involvement. Such a sediment is rich in a mixture of all types of casts and inflammatory cells. It was believed at one time to be pathognomonic of lupus nephritis; however, it is observed also in a wide variety of other actively progressive nephritic disorders.

ELEMENTS UNRELATED TO THE PATHOLOGY OF THE URINARY SYSTEM

It is not an infrequent problem to be confronted by material in the urine sediment which does not originate in the urinary tract or is difficult to identify. A variety of fibers are commonly seen, such as bits of thread or paper. Hair is a common finding. On occasion the material defies identification.

TISSUE IN THE URINE

On rare occasions small clumps of renal tissue may appear in the urine sediment. This material can be identified because of its large size and because it is composed of many cells. Precise identification of such material is highly desirable so that an accurate diagnosis can be made. Transfer of the observed material to appropriate fixatives may help to preserve it so that ultimate histologic evaluation can be performed. This is especially important if the tissue, for example, represents renal papillar elements which may suggest the presence of papillary necrosis.

SUPRAVITAL CYTODIAGNOSTIC STAIN FOR URINARY SEDIMENTS

Sternheimer (59) reported the following:

A mixture of aqueous solutions of National fast blue (formerly Allied Chemical Corp., now Matheson, Coleman, and Bell, Norwood, Ohio 45212), a copper phthalocyanine dye, and Pyronin B (Matheson, Coleman, and Bell), a red xanthine dye, when added to fresh urinary sediment supravitally stains benign or malignant cells and the various types of casts and their inclusions. Stain facilitates identification of the formed elements and particularly aids in the differentiation of polymorphonuclear leukocytes from lymphocytes, histiocytes, plasma cells, and renal tubular cells. A variable staining of casts and their inclusions has been observed. Tumor cells may be recognized by nuclear abnormalities or in case of hyperchromatic tendency, by a very rapid and early uptake of dye preceding that of the surrounding cells. This staining method is rapid and simple enough for routine urinalysis and screening procedures.

6 Clinical Screening

Today virtually all routine urine testing is done by dipstick. There are dipsticks available to perform a wide array of qualitative tests on urine (Table 6–1). Quantitative information for these constituents requires additional procedures. The classical chemical procedure reagents for protein, glucose, bile, etc., are incorporated as a dried residue on a paper or plastic stick which is then immersed in fresh urine. A characteristic color develops which is compared to a chart of various colors showing quantitative amounts.

USAGE AND COMPARISONS OF DIFFERENT METHODS

The stick or test tapes for sugar determination are specific for glucose since they use a glucose oxidase procedure, but they fail to detect the presence of other sugars. They may miss such conditions as galactosemia and hereditary fructose intolerance, both of which may be lethal in a newborn and may represent serious illnesses in older children. The approach for detecting any reducing substance may be preferable in a newborn (see Ch. 15, Generalized Metabolic Derangement). All reducing substances are determined by the Clinitest table.*

*Manufactured by Ames Company, Division of Miles Laboratories, Inc., Elkhart, Indiana 46514)

TABLE 6-1. RAPID REAGENT TESTS FOR ROUTINE AND SPECIAL URINALYSES.

Reagent test	Substances determined	Technique
Multistix* Reagent strips	pH, albumin, glucose ketones, bilirubin, hemoglobin or myoglobin, and urobilinogen	Use fresh, uncentrifuged urine. Preservatives may be added. Dip reagent strip in specimen, remove and compare each reagent area with corresponding color chart on bottle label at the number of seconds specified.
Chemstrip 8**	Nitrite, pH, albumin, glucose, ketones, urobilinogen, bilirubin, hemoglobin or myoglobin	Same as above
Bili-labstix*	pH, albumin, glucose, ketones, bilirubin, hemoglobin or myoglobin	Same as above
Labstix*	pH, albumin, glucose, ketones, hemoglobin or myoglobin	Same as above
Hema-combistix*	pH, albumin, glucose, hemoglobin or myoglobin	Same as above
Combistix*	pH, albumin, and glucose	Same as above
Uristix*	Albumin and glucose	Same as above
Albustix*	Albumin	Same as above
Hemastix*	Hemoglobin or myoglobin	Same as above
Urobilistix*	Urobilinogen	Same as above, but preferably using a 2-hour urine specimen collected in early afternoon (between 2 and 4 P.M.)
Microstix*	Bacteriuria	Dip Culture-reagent strip in specimen for 5 sec, remove, read nitrite test area after 30 sec. Insert and seal strip in sterilized plastic pouch provided, incubate for 18–24 hours. Compare color densities on total and gram-negative culture pads with chart provided, without removing strip from pouch. Incinerate pouch with strip still sealed inside.
Ictotest*	Bilirubin	Place 5 drops of urine on the special mat. Cover with the reagent tablet. Flow 2 drops of water onto tablet. Compare the color reaction with the color chart.

TABLE 6-1. RAPID REAGENT TESTS FOR ROUTINE AND SPECIAL URINALYSIS *(continued)*

Reagent test	Substances determined	Technique
Diastix*	Glucose	Use fresh, uncentrifuged urine. Do not use preservative containing formaldehyde. Dip reagent strip in specimen 2 sec., remove, and compare with color chart on bottle label.
Testape***	Glucose	Same as above
Ketostix*	Ketones (principally acetoacetic acid)	Same as above, but urine must be at room temperature at time of testing.
Keto-diastix*	Glucose and ketones (principally acetoacetic acid)	Same as above for Diastix and Ketostix.
Clinitest*	Reducing substances, including sugars	Add Clinitest tablet to test tube containing mixture of 5 drops of urine and 10 drops of water. Spontaneous boiling occurs; after it stops, compare color in tube with color chart.
Phenistix*	Phenylpyruvic acid (phenylketonuria, or PKU)	Use fresh, uncentrifuged urine. Dip reagent strip in specimen, remove, and compare with color chart on bottle label.

*The Ames Co., Division of Miles Laboratories Inc.
**Bio-dynamics/bmc, Division of Boehringer & Mannheim, GmbH
***Smith, Kline and French Laboratories
(Adapted from Modern Urinalysis, Elkhart, The Ames Co., 1974)

The stick test for protein is specific for albumin. This is of special importance when large amounts of light-chain proteins of the alpha or kappa type Bence–Jones proteins appear in the relative absence of albumin. The stick would not detect these chemicals; however, a denaturation procedure for protein, such as the use of sulfasalicylic acid, would detect the protein (see Ch 10, Protein).

7 Urinary pH

The term **pH** is an expression of the hydrogen ion (H^+) concentration of a solution. The pH value of a urine sample thus reflects the concentration of H^+ in that solution. An important function of the kidney in part is the regulation of the pH of body fluids. The maintenance of a constant pH in the body fluids is critical to the well-being of the individual.

The kidney is able to regulate the H^+ content of the urine over a wide range. Thereby, in appropriate situations, large amounts of H^+ will appear in the urine; this urine will have a pH of less than 7 (the more H^+, the lower the pH), and is referred to as an acid or acidic urine. The lowest urine pH (highest H^+ content) which can be produced by the normal kidney is 4.5. On the other hand, the kidney may need to conserve H^+ and excrete a urine with a very low concentration of H^+; this urine will have a pH of greater than 7 (the less H^+, the higher the pH) and is referred to as an alkaline or basic urine. The highest urine pH the normal kidney can produce (the lowest H^+ content) is 8 (5,6,42,52).

Interpretation of the urine pH should be done in context with internal and external factors which may mediate the pH of body fluids (12a). It is only with a knowledge of this circumstance that a proper interpretation can be made. If the urine pH is greater than 8, this signifies that bacteria which are able to degrade urea to ammonia are present in the formed urine. Ammonia combines with H^+ or water to form ammonium hydroxide, a substance which removes H^+ from a solution. There is no substance spontaneously formed which could inappropriately reduce the urine pH. A urine pH of less than 4.5 would reflect the presence of an acid in the urine collection container.

METHODS

The usual method for measurement of pH utilizes the dipstick or indicator papers. These papers have various dye indicators impregnated into the paper and exhibit a color change specific to the pH of the urine. The pH range of these papers and the reasonable accuracy of pH change make them satisfactory for pH measurement of freshly voided urine.

A glass electrode coupled with an electrometer is the most accurate method for measurement of pH. If the electrode and electrometer apparatus is properly calibrated, using standard solutions which have pHs above and below the measured pH, an accurate form of measurement is obtained. Measurement of pH to the tenths of units is more than adequate for the most exacting clinical purpose (4,12,28,32,34,58).

Precise measurements require that the urine be freshly collected and free of bacteria. Bacteria can degrade urea to ammonia even in the bladder and thereby decrease the pH of the formed urine. Should any delay occur between the time of collection and the time of analysis, the urine should be drawn into a glass syringe from which all air bubbles have been removed. The syringe should be capped and kept chilled in an ice slush. At the time of measurement, the temperature of the urine should be measured and appropriate corrections of the instrumentation made to correct for temperature of the urine at the time of measurement.

8 Glucose and Other Sugars

Glucose appears in the urine in significant amounts when the kidneys' reabsorptive threshold for glucose has been exceeded.

The concentration of glucose in the plasma and in the initial glomerular filtrate is equal (Fig. 8-1) (66). For example, when the plasma glucose (P_g) equals 100 mg/dl and the glomerular filtrate glucose (U_g) equals 100 mg/dl just beyond the glomerular capillary membrane and if 150 liters of glomerular filtrate are initially formed in 24 hours, then U_g multiplied by 150 liters equals 150,000 mg, or 150 g, of glucose which is filtered. In most instances, virtually all of this 150 g is reabsorbed by tubular mechanisms. As a result, little, if any, glucose appears in the urine.

Two factors, however, may lead to the appearance of glucose in the urine. The plasma glucose concentration may exceed the reabsorptive capacity of the kidney, or the reabsorptive capacity of the kidney may be reduced (40). The reabsorptive capacity for glucose is usually exceeded when the plasma glucose exceeds 150-180 mg/dl. Any event which causes hyperglycemia, generally in excess of 180 mg/dl, will result in the appearance of glucose in the urine. The differential diagnosis of hyperglycemia includes disease categories and physiologic states.

Sustained, persistent hyperglycemia in excess of the threshold reabsorptive capacity can result in the excretion of large amounts of glucose in the urine. Over a period of 24 hours, up to 300 g glucose may be excreted when the plasma glucose level is very elevated. The glucose molecule acts as a nonreabsorbable substance (similar to mannitol) and creates an obligatory need for water as well as electrolytes, hence promoting an

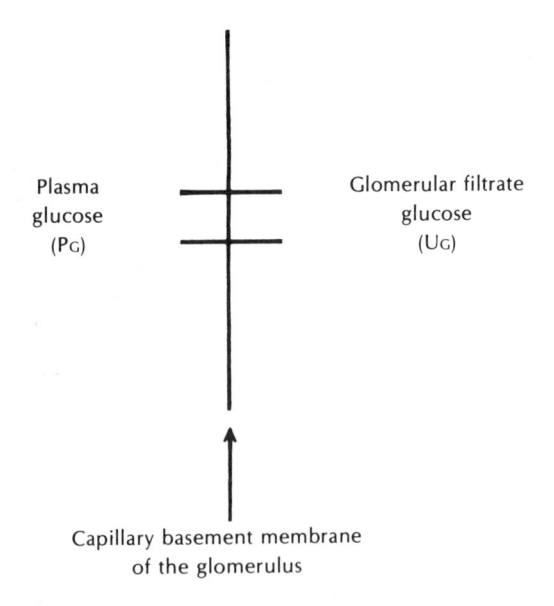

Fig. 8–1. Concentration of glucose in the plasma is equal to that of the glomerular filtrate.

increased excretion of water and electrolytes. The diuretic effect of persistent glycosuria can be substantial.

Glucose may also appear in the urine if the reabsorptive threshold for glucose is depressed. As a result, even with a normal or slightly elevated plasma glucose concentration, glucose may appear in the urine. Depression of the reabsorptive threshold for glucose may be congenital or acquired. Acquired glycosuria with normal blood glucose levels is often seen in patients with tubular damage and in some patients with nephrosis (19,40).

In order to interpret the significance of glucose in the urine it is necessary to measure blood sugar levels simultaneously. In addition, the urine sample should be collected within the same time frame as the plasma sample. To obtain a carefully collected sample, the patient should first void, emptying the bladder; then after an appropriate interval of time has elapsed (1–2 hours) the patient should be asked to void again. It is the glucose measurement of this sample that can be correlated with a blood sugar measurement obtained during the midpoint of the collection.

METHOD OF MEASUREMENT

The traditional method for measuring glucose is based upon its property as a reducing agent. Because many substances appearing in the urine can serve as reducing substances, such an analysis is not specific for glucose. However, the ease of measurement, joined with the knowledge of those substances which give a false-positive reaction for glucose (Table 8-1), permit the use of this method in the evaluation of urine glucose.

To determine the presence of a copper-reducing substance, mix the urine with Benedict's solution. With heat, color will change from blue to orange if a reducing substance is present (41). This same type of reaction is the basis for the Clinitest tablet test. In this instance the reagent is in a dry form which is dissolved when it comes in contact with urine.

A specific test for glucose utilizes the enzyme glucose oxidase (62). False-positive tests only occur with hypochlorite and peroxide, both of which do not appear in urine. However, two substances, ascorbic acid and ketones, which appear in the urine may interfere with the reaction and produce a false-negative test.

The most convenient form of glucose oxidase testing is the dipstick or tape. Both are very sensitive indicators of the presence of glucose in the urine (15). Dilution of the urine can be performed to obtain a semi-quantitative result. Alternatively, the Clinitest tablet or Benedicts's solution, both of which are less sensitive but cover a wider range of glucose concentrations, can be utilized (See Table 16-1).

Quantitative measurement of glucose is sometimes necessary. This is especially the case when the clinician is attempting to regulate insulin

TABLE 8-1. INTERFERING SUBSTANCES IN TESTS FOR GLUCOSURIA

Copper reduction tests
False-positive reactions

Ascorbic acid	Phenol*
Salicylates*	Turpentine
Cephalothin	Glucosamine
Creatinine	Streptomycin
Uric acid	Isoniazid
Penicillin	p-Aminosalicylic acid*
Ampicillin	Demethylchlortetracycline
Chloral hydrate*	Formaldehyde
Paraldehyde*	Aminopyrine*
Camphor	Nalidixic acid
Methol*	

Enzyme tests

False-negative	*False-positive*
Ascorbic acid	Hypochlorite
Ketones	Peroxide

*Excreted as glucuronide, a reducing agent.
(Modified from Wilson DM: Minn Med 58(1):9–17, 1975)

requirements of a diabetic patient. Quantitative measurement of the urine glucose is also necessary when the tubular reabsorption of glucose is measured. Urine samples obtained on quantitative analysis should be refrigerated immediately after collection. Preservatives should not be added because they will interfere with oxidase reaction. The quantitative analysis of urine can utilize the same systems as those for plasma determinations if appropriate dilution is made.

9 Ketones

A variety of factors leads to the development of ketonuria. Almost invariably the basic problem is an absolute or relative deficiency of insulin.

The ketone bodies, acetone, diacetic acid (acetoacetic acid), and β-hydroxybutyric acid, apparently originate primarily in the liver in disorders such as starvation and diabetes mellitus. In these conditions little glycogen is available for energy so that fat, which has as its by-products the ketone bodies, must be utilized for energy. These compounds are slightly acidic and in very high concentrations may contribute to clinical acidosis (2).

Only acetoacetic acid and acetone are measured by conventional methodology. These substances are readily filtered by the glomerulus and are subjected to little, if any, reabsorption by the tubules of the kidney. As a consequence, these ketone substances appear readily in urine. Their presence in the urine implies that their concentration in the serum is elevated as well.

It should be recognized that large amounts of β-hydroxybutyric acid may be present in both blood and urine and yet not detected by the conventional nitroprusside test. Diabetic ketoacidosis is frequently accompanied by a large accumulation of these compounds, a condition that may be more significant than the measurement of the acetoacetate and acetone might suggest. However, the nitroprusside test is recommended because it is sensitive, easy to perform, and positive for either acetone or acetoacetic acid. The same clinical significance is attached to both substances; and at the time of testing, the ketone may exist in either or both forms. Therefore, a test that detects either has greater application than does the test that measures only one form of the ketone. It is of academic interest only to demonstrate that, in a particular type of ketonuria, the percentage of acetoacetic acid is higher than that of acetone or vice versa. It is also very rare that ketonemia ever produces a ketonuria that is exclusively due to β-hydroxybutyric acid; a nitroprusside test on the urine amply demonstrates the ketonuria without the difficult test for β-hydroxybutyric acid.

In using the nitroprusside procedure, it must be realized that a small amount of acetoacetic acid (2 mg/dl of urine) promptly produces a purple color but that acetone produces a similar purple color only after several minutes, even when present in much heavier concentrations (30 mg/dl of sample). For added sensitivity of detecting ketonuria, it is recommended that freshly voided urine be used and that testing be performed before the acetoacetic acid has been converted to acetone. The test can be performed with nitroprusside reagent strips, such as Ketostix.* If the commercially prepared reagent strips are unavailable, either Lange's or Rothera's test can be performed, either of which is easy and reliable.

PRINCIPLE OF THE TEST

Both acetoacetic acid and its more stable decomposition product, acetone, form a purple complex with a saturated solution of nitroprusside when overlaid with ammonia. A similarly colored complex is produced in the reagent strips prepared commercially. Knowledge of the chemistry of this reaction is very limited and prevents any comprehensive consideration of the causes for a positive test. There appear to be very few causes, however, for a false-positive result such as is observed with many of the other tests performed upon urine, including the ferric chloride test for acetoacetic acid. In general, it may be concluded that the only cause for a positive nitroprusside test on the urine is ketonuria. The fact that both acetone and acetoacetic acid are readily volatilized by heat offers an easy way to verify a positive test as being due to ketones (2).

TECHNIQUES

Two procedures to test for acetone or acetoacetic acid are Lange's and Rothera's methods. Lange's method is as follows:

1. To about 5 ml urine in a test tube, add five drops of glacial acetic acid.
2. Add a few drops of saturated aqueous solution of sodium nitroprusside.
3. Overlay with 1–2 ml ammonia water to develop purple color.

*Manufactured by Ames Company. Elkhart, Indiana 46514

4. Read and report as negative, weakly positive, or strongly positive.

Rothera's method is as follows:

1. To about 5 ml urine in a test tube, add approximately 1 g ammonium sulfate.
2. Add two or three drops of saturated aqueous solution of sodium nitroprusside.
3. Overlay with 1–2 ml of ammonia water.
4. Read and report as described in Lange's method.

VERIFICATION TEST

Perform the following steps for increased specificity to verify that the positive reaction seen in the nitroprusside test is due to ketones.

1. To one volume of urine, an aliquot of which has exhibited a positive nitroprusside reaction, add one volume of water.
2. Boil down to one volume.
3. Perform the nitroprusside test upon the residue.
4. A negative test indicates that ketones gave the original positive test, while a residue that again gives a positive test indicates some other cause for the positive results.

The normal blood level for ketones in the postprandial condition is reported to be 0.1–1.0 mg/dl in acetone equivalence. The ketones exist, however, almost entirely as acetoacetic and β-hydroxybutyric acids. The 24-hour urinary output of ketones is under 20 mg for a normal person on a regular diet. This urinary concentration (1.3 mg/dl) is inadequate to give a positive nitroprusside test even though all of the ketones eliminated were in the most detectable form. (For example, acetoacetic acid at a concentration of 2 mg/dl gives a faintly positive test, but 30 mg/dl of acetone is required for a positive result.)

In cases of prolonged starvation or severe diabetic acidosis, the ketone level in the blood may increase manyfold, and the 24-hour urinary excretion increases tremendously, with values as high as 100 g/24 hours being reported (14,17).

REAGENT STRIPS

If no purple discoloration develops within 15 sec after the strip is moistened with urine, a negative reaction is reported. A positive reaction is reported as small, moderate, or large, depending upon the intensity of the purple produced within 15 sec.

Lange's or Rothera's tests are ring tests; a positive result is characterized by a purple interface developing between the ammonia overlay and the nitroprusside-impregnated urine below. As in other ring tests, the diameter of the zone of reaction of a positive test is more closely related to the care used in adding the overlay material than it is to the quantity of substance present. Therefore, it is unwarranted to try to quantitate the amount of ketones present in the urine any more precisely than to report the test results as negative, weakly positive (trace), or strongly positive as gauged by the intensity and amount of purple color developed.

10 Protein

Protein is one of the most important and often pathologically significant determinations in the routine urinalysis, and quantitative examinations for proteins should be done on all specimens. Proteinuria is usually an important indicator of renal damage.

The quantity and composition of the proteins in urine vary widely in the pathophysiologic states of renal disease (39). For example, hemolysis of blood may produce hemoglobin in the urine; acute glomerulonephritis leads to albumin in the urine; multiple myeloma may result in Bence–Jones proteinuria; and tubular necrosis may produce a mixture of intracellular proteins appearing in the urine.

MECHANISMS OF PROTEINURIA

The glomerular filtrate contains a very low concentration of protein. In animal studies where techniques have permitted the sampling of the glomerular filtrate, the amount of protein which passes through the glomerular membrane is very low and consists generally of low-molecular-weight proteins (molecules smaller than hemoglobin and albumin). These substances are probably reabsorbed in the proximal tubule so that the final urine contains less than 150 mg protein in 24 hours.

Proteinuria greater than 150 mg/24 hours may occur if 1) a defect in the glomerular capillary membrane permits the escape of high-molecular-weight proteins into the glomerular filtrate or 2) a defect exists in the reabsorptive mechanisms in the proximal tubule. Often defects in both mechanisms coexist.

Proteinuria of glomerular origin may occur with a normal appearing glomerular capillary membrane by light and electron microscopy criteria or may occur with severe histologic abnormalities of the glomerulus.

Causes of glomerular proteinuria include the following:

1. Nil-change disease (minimal change disease)—lipoid nephrosis
2. Glomerulonephritis

   Membranous glomerulonephritis
   Proliferative glomerulonephritis
   Membranoproliferative glomerulonephritis
   Congenital and familiar nephrosis
   Amyloid disease of the kidney
   Diabetes
   Systemic lupus erythematosus
   Renal venous thrombosis
   Hypersensitivity reaction to drugs
   Toxic effect of drugs on the glomerular membrane
   Pregnancy
   Collagen vascular disease
   Schönlein–Henoch purpura
   Wegener's granulomatosis

Glomerular proteinuria consists of high-molecular-weight proteins (greater than 60,000 daltons) with albumin being a prominent and occasionally exclusive component. The excretion of these proteins may barely exceed the normal protein excretion (150 mg/day) or may reach levels exceeding 40 g/day.

Protein of tubular origin rarely exceeds 1 g in 24 hours and consists of a low-molecular-weight protein (less than 60,000 daltons). Tubular proteinuria may reflect the filtration of a low-molecular-weight compound in large amounts (such as kappa or lambda chain—Bence–Jones proteins) or may represent damage to the tubular reabsorptive membranes which are now unable to reabsorb normally filtered protein.

Differential diagnosis of tubular proteinuria includes the following:

1. Congenital tubulopathies

   Primary renal tubular acidosis
   Multiple defects of tubular functions
   Chronic hypokalemia and hyperkaluria
   Oculocerebrorenal dystrophy
   Nephrogenic diabetes insipidus
   Glomerular tubular proteinuria and related conditions

2. Systemic diseases with tubular defects—leukemia
3. Acute renal insufficiency
4. Interstitial nephritis
5. Nephritis of unknown origin

   Nephrophthisis
   Alport's syndrome

6. Balkan nephropathy

MEASUREMENT OF PROTEIN IN URINE

The usual method of measuring protein in urine utilizes the dipstick. The dipstick is especially sensitive to albumin and is based on the fact that tetrabromphenol blue changes to yellow in the absence of protein when buffered at a pH of 3. With protein present, the color becomes a green blue at the same pH. This colorimetric test is quite sensitive to albumin, giving a positive reaction to as little as 20–25 mg/dl. It is less sensitive to globulins and fibrinogen, requiring a considerably higher concentration of these proteins to produce the same extent of color change. It is not sensitive to Bence–Jones protein.

Another method commonly utilized to measure protein in the urinalysis laboratory is that of precipitation. Plasma proteins are completely soluble in aqueous solutions through a wide range of pHs, and there are many different tests for the detection of protein in the urine based on the precipitation of these proteins out of the urine solution. These tests make the protein insoluble, resulting in a white flocculent precipitant suspension. This insoluble state may be created by heat coagulation, salting-out techniques, or by the action of so-called alkaloid salt such as sulfosalicylic acid, phosphomolybdic–phosphotungstic acid, and trichloroacetic acid. Proteins are less stable and more susceptible to precipitating agents when at the pH of their isoelectric point. While the isoelectric point is not the same for all proteins, most are at a low pH, which explains why the time-honored heat and acid test for urinary protein is still acceptable. The test to be used is chosen by the pathologist and medical technologist with consideration of the number of tests being given daily and the available instrumentation. The sulfosalicylic acid method of precipitation is favored by many since the time-consuming heating process is eliminated.

For those laboratories choosing to employ one or more of the conventional patient tests either the heat and acid test or the sulfosalicylic acid test is recommended. The various overlay ring tests are not recommended since they are more time consuming and do not lend themselves as well to any semiquantitative method of reporting.

HEAT AND ACID TEST

The heat and acid test is carried out as follows:

1. Heat a few milliliters of centrifuged urine to boiling in a test tube.
2. Add a few drops of acid (acetic 5% or concentrated nitric acid). The acid is used for two purposes, to dissolve any phosphates or carbonates that may be the cause of a white cloudiness and to lower the pH to a point near the isoelectric point of proteins and thus make the heat-coagulated proteins more insoluble.
3. Read and report in accordance with degree of cloudiness observed.

SULFOSALICYLIC ACID TEST

The sulfosalicylic acid test may be used as an aqueous 20% solution, although lower concentrations have been used, or as Exton's qualitative reagent, which is sulfosalicylic acid 5% in a solution of sodium sulfate (8.8 g/dl). Proceed as follows:

1. Add a few drops of the sulfosalicylic acid 20% solution to a few milliliters of filtered or centrifuged urine. (Add an equal volume of Exton's if this reagent is used.)
2. Remove the cloudiness produced by either urates or proteoses, such as the Bence–Jones protein, from consideration by heating. Urate clouding disappears upon warming, and proteose clouding disappears upon boiling.
3. Read and record the degree of cloudiness.

TEST REPORTS

It has become a practice, with merit, to report all qualitative chemical tests that are a part of the routine urinalysis in a semiquantitative manner by grading the intensity of the reaction.

REAGENT STRIP TEST

A semiquantification of urinary protein can be made on the basis of the intensity of the green blue discoloration produced in the bromphenol blue indicator. The manufacturer provides a chart with a grading of the nuances of color that permits a report ranging from negative to a 4+ protein concentration. These grades are as follows:

```
Negative = under 10 mg/dl
Trace    = 15–25 mg/dl
1+       = 30 mg/dl
```

2+ = 100 mg/dl
3+ = 300 mg/dl
4+ = 1000 (or more) mg/dl

PRECIPITATION METHODS

Quantitative estimation of urinary proteins can be made from an evaluation of the intensity or quantity of precipitate formed regardless of the precipitating agent used. Custom has entrenched the method of recording the quantity of precipitate formed in degrees of positivity of the test, *i.e.*, the number of pluses, from one to four, serving to quantify the concentration of protein in the urine.

There is little agreement on the exact quantitative meaning of a report that indicates, for example, that the protein is 3+ in the specimen. This arises from the fact that different test procedures produce variable quantities of floccules with the same protein concentration, and observers may not always agree on the degree of opalescence required for a given number of pluses.

In spite of these variables, this method of quantification is quite valuable to the clinician, particularly on serial determination (36). Actually, the method becomes fairly precise in the hands of a technologist who performs a large number of tests daily using a single method. It is for this reason that it seems desirable to ascribe some quantitative value to the commonly used plus values with the full realization that these are only approximations. Reports that are negative indicate no cloudiness (zero protein). A trace (±) indicates a cloudiness so faint that a dark background is needed for detection (up to 0.03 g/dl). One plus (1+) indicates cloudiness distinct against a black background but barely visible against a light background (0.03–0.05 g/dl); 2+, cloudiness which is granular appearing and distinct even with a light background (0.05–0.20 g/dl); 3+, cloudiness which is floccular and heavy (0.2–0.5 g/dl); 4+, cloudiness which is dense and shows large individual floccules (over 0.5 g/dl). If 3 g/dl or more is present, the urine solidifies upon boiling.

Quantitative measurement of protein can be done by a variety of techniques as shown by Pesce (45) (Table 10–1). The Kingsbury–Clark method can be utilized for developing a quantitative test; it involves the precipitation of urine proteins with sulfosalicylic acid 3% and a turbidimetric reading on a photometer. For this reason, the urine should first be centrifuged to eliminate cloudiness due to formed elements. After 2.5 ml urine supernatant and 7.5 ml acid are mixed in a tube, the mixture is allowed to stand 3–5 min. The percent of transmittance is read at 550 nm and converted to mg/dl of protein from the calibration curve. When the

TABLE 10-1. QUANTITATIVE PROTEIN DETERMINATION METHODS

Method	Principle	Comment
Kjeldahl	Chemical; measures nitrogen content of protein	Standard reference method; for urinary protein all nonprotein nitrogen must be removed, which may greatly exceed the protein nitrogen
Biuret	Chemical; copper complexes with peptide bonds in alkaline solution	Measures protein and peptides in native urine, with some interference from urea and colored metabolites; a good method, but inaccurate at low protein concentrations, because it requires concentration of protein
Folin–Lowry	Chemical; biuret and redox reaction; redox reaction very sensitive to tyrosyl and tryptophanyl residues	Sensitive method; strong interference by compounds such as uric acid, which require precipitation of protein and washing to remove them; reference standards a problem, as tyrosyl and tryptophanyl residues of proteins vary widely
Precipitation (sulfosalicylic acid, trichloroacetic acid, or phosphotungstic acid)	Protein precipitates; measure scattered light or amount of precipitate formed	Inaccurate, since not all proteins form same type of precipitate in terms of volume space/mg protein; some false-positive reactions; some types of proteinuria may be missed (e.g., small molecular weight glycoproteins)
Heat and acetic acid	Protein precipitates at pH 5 upon heating	
Dye binding (Combustix)	Proteins, especially albumin, bind dye, thereby changing color of dye	Interference from metabolic products which also compete for the dye binding sites; not all proteins, particularly Bence–Jones, bind the dye; method more specific for albumin than any other protein
Refractive index	Physical; protein has higher refractive index than water	Salts, metabolic products present in large and variable accounts; thus of no value to measure protein
Specific gravity	Physical; protein is denser than water	Salts and metabolic products outweigh protein concentration; no value as measurement method

(Pesce AJ: Nephron 13:93–104, 1974)

percent of transmittance reading exceeds the upper values of the calibration curve prepared using bovine serum albumin, the test must be repeated using a dilution of the supernatant so that results fall within the range of calibration (Table 10–2).

When a heavily colored urine is being tested, it is sometimes necessary to make a colorblank using the appropriate amount of supernatant and substituting water for acid.

Determination of total protein on a 24-hour urine specimen is done by this same method. The urine volume must first be measured. Calculations for total protein are done by moving the decimal point two places to the left for the total volume of urine and multiplying by the mg/dl protein.

For example:

> Total volume (TV) = 1600 ml
> and the protein value is found to be 42 mg/dl
> Total protein (TP) = 16 × 42 = 672 mg protein/24 hours

Detectable amounts of protein are not normal in random specimens; 0–10 mg/dl readings are reported as negative; 10–20 mg/dl are reported as a trace; values of up to 150 mg/24 hours are considered normal by the authors.

ORTHOSTATIC PROTEINURIA

Detection of orthostatic proteinuria requires special procedures for collection. Orthostatic proteinuria occurs in an individual only when that person is standing but not when recumbent. This type of proteinuria is further increased in the exaggerated lordotic position. Proteinuria only in the upright position is in general not associated with histologic disease in the kidney, is a benign finding, and therefore serves as a test to distinguish types of proteinuria. While this procedure can be done in a variety of ways, the following is one alternative.

TABLE 10-2. DILUTION FOR QUANTITATIVE URINE PROTEIN DETERMINATION

Dilution	Supernatant	Acid
None	2.5 ml	7.5 ml
5×	0.5	9.5
10×	0.25	9.75
25×	0.1	9.9
50×	0.05	9.95

SUPINE URINE

The patient is kept in bed in the recumbent position (preferably during the night hours for a 12-hour period). The patient may stand or sit to void but in all other respects is to remain recumbent. That urine is then submitted as a 12-hour sample for measurement of protein.

UPRIGHT URINE

The patient is then asked to be up and about during the following 12 hours for as much time as possible. Particularly, the patient is not to assume the supine position but rather may sit or, preferably, stand for as much time as can be tolerated. That urine specimen is then submitted as the upright urine and protein over the 12-hour period is measured.

INTERPRETATION

The patient with orthostatic proteinuria should not excrete any protein of significance in the supine position, *i.e.*, less than 75 mg over the 12-hour period of collection, and should excrete a significant amount of protein in the upright position (greater than 75 mg). It is not uncommon for patients with persistent proteinuria to have some increase in the amount of protein excretion while in the upright position. This does not, however, indicate orthostatic proteinuria in the true sense.

INTERFERENCES AND FALSE TESTS

With dipstick testing, false-positive tests may occur with alkaline, highly buffered urines. Contaminating quaternary ammonium compounds may also give false-positive tests, as may certain drugs. With Kingsbury–Clark testing, proteinlike reactions occur in urine from patients who have recently received radiopaque solutions for certain x-ray procedures, *e.g.*, intravenous pyelogram. Other false-positive reactions may be due to urine turbidity, color, heavy mucus, proteoses, and large numbers of WBCs.

Young (67) has compiled an extensive list of drugs and their effects on clinical laboratory tests. Information is derived from many scientific and medical journals. Several thousand interfering substances are included. Individual copies may be obtained from the American Association of Clinical Chemists, 1725 K Street, N.W., Washington, D.C. 20006.

PREPARING A PROTEIN SPECTROPHOTOMETER CURVE

A spectrophotometric standard curve should be prepared for protein every 6 months when the protein quality control value changes (as with a new lot number of quality control) or when weekly quality control indicates variation outside the limits of acceptance for the existing curve.

In preparing the curve, the quality control product *e.g.*, Urintrol*, is treated exactly as a specimen. A control sample with the value of the quality control product is prepared. Serial dilutions are prepared and their concentrations calculated to determine other points on the curve.

1. Place 2.5 ml of the control product in a test tube. This tube contains the undiluted control.
2. Place 2.5 ml of a 1:2 dilution in the second tube.
3. Place 2.5 ml of a 1:4 dilution in the third tube.
4. Place 2.5 ml of a 1:8 dilution in the fourth tube.
5. After dilutions are made, each tube will contain 2.5 ml of the proper dilution.
6. Add 7.5 ml sulfosalicylic acid to the four tubes.
7. Mix each tube; let stand 3–5 min and read the percent of transmission (%T).
8. Plot %T versus calculated concentration in mg/dl on semilog paper; draw the curve (passing through the point of 0 mg/dl and 100%T). Since the linearity cannot always be assumed, extending the curve past the highest point of known concentration is not advisable. Protein values higher than this concentration must be diluted.

An example for plotting the curve is demonstrated in Figure 10–1. In this case, the quality control value is 100 mg/dl and the %T reading of the control is set at 100 mg/dl. Dilutions are set up as follows: 1:2, 50 mg/dl; 1:4, 25 mg/dl; 1:8, 25 mg/dl. This material is then plotted on a graph as shown (Fig. 10–1). Specimens of unknown concentrations can now be prepared and their %T determined on the spectrophotometer. Reading these %T values from the curve, the concentrations may then be found (53).

BENCE–JONES PROTEIN

The dipstick method for urine screening is sensitive primarily to albumin; as a consequence, Bence-Jones proteinuria can be missed. These proteins do not react with the tetrabromphenol blue reagent in the dipstick. These

*Manufactured by Harleco, Philadelphia, Pennsylvania

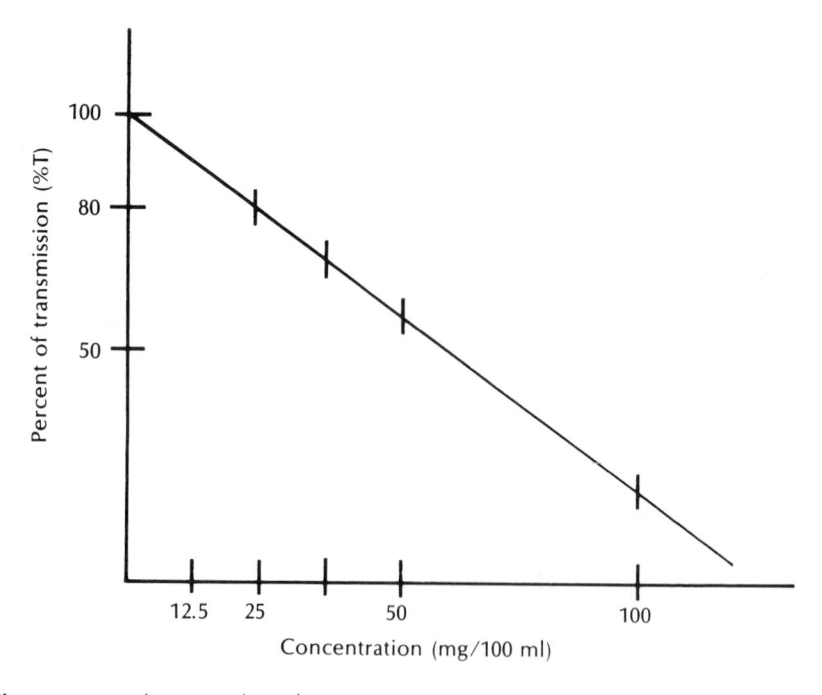

Fig. 10–1. Quality control graph.

substances, however, are detected by the various precipitation methods. It therefore is important that the urine of any patient who is suspected of having Bence-Jones proteinuria be checked with a precipitation method. A point of differential diagnosis can be established if the dipstick test shows a slight degree of proteinuria and if the precipitation test shows a great deal of proteinuria. This protein is a substance which originates from plasma cells in the bone marrow and other sites. Its molecular weight is approximately 40,000 daltons, and it is filtered by the glomerular capillary membrane. This substance may appear in the urine in surprisingly large quantities. Its continued filtration has a deleterious effect in overall renal function.

Bence–Jones protein has two unusual properties: 1) it will precipitate on heating to 40°–70° C (optimum 56° C), and 2) it redissolves at temperatures of 100° C. These properties may be utilized in screening urines.

Effersoe and Tidstrom (22) reported a simple salting-out procedure for Bence–Jones protein using a phosphate buffer solution. They reported a 50% greater number of positive results (19 out of 21 cases of known mutiple myeloma) than they observed with the usual temperature of flocculation procedure (only 13 positives of the 21 cases). Ritzmann *et al.* (49), reporting on the fallibility of classification of myeloma proteins, indicate that efforts to diagnose multiple myeloma by demonstration of a protein that is insoluble only at about 60° C leaves much to be desired as a screening test. Diagnosis of multiple myeloma may be difficult even when the patient's proteins are characterized through studies using electrophoresis, ultracentrifugation, and immunodiffusion techniques. At the present time, immunoprotein electrophoresis is considered to be the best screening test for myeloma.

A variety of methods are available for detection of Bence-Jones protein. One procedure is as follows:

1. Screen a random urine specimen for protein using the Kingsbury–Clark method. When protein is negative, report Bence–Jones as negative. When protein is found, continue.
2. Mix 4 ml centrifuged urine and 1 ml sodium acetate buffer, pH 4.9. Place in a 56° C water bath for 10–15 min; examine for turbidity or precipitation.
3. If precipitation occurs, remove supernatant fluid and resuspend the precipitate in 2 ml sulfosalicylic acid 3%. When the test has become turbid, centrifuge to get a buttonlike precipitate at the bottom of the tube.
4. Heat to boiling for 5–10 min while observing the precipitate. A precipitate that dissolves is considered to be Bence–Jones protein. A precipitate that does not dissolve at 100° C is reported as negative.
5. Alternatively, the urine can be mixed with the toluene sulfonic acid (TSA) reagent, and a positive flocculation would be strongly suggestive of Bence–Jones proteinuria.

The procedure for toluene sulfonic acid screening test for Bence–Jones protein is as follows (13):

Technique

1. Pipette 2 ml clear, fresh urine into a test tube.
2. Add 1 ml TSA reagent by allowing the reagent to flow slowly (15–30 sec) down the side of the tube.
3. Flick the tube with a finger.
4. A precipitate occurring within 5 min is a positive test for Bence–Jones protein, *i.e.*, free light chains.

Reagents

1. 12 g p-toluene sulfonic acid
2. 100 ml acetic acid

This method is capable of detecting as little as 0.03 mg/ml of Bence–Jones protein. Albumin does not precipitate in concentrations as high as 25 g/dl. Normal α, β, and γ-globulins will precipitate with TSA reagent but only when present in concentrations greater than 1 mg/ml urine. In general, this test is more sensitive and reliable than the heat and precipitation test. A positive TSA test does not make the diagnosis of myeloma or any other plasma cell dyscrasia; it only indicates the presence of excessive amounts of free light chains in the urine. Cellulose acetate electrophoresis and immunoelectrophoresis are necessary to characterize the proteinuria accurately.

11 Addis Count

The Addis count is only used occasionally at the present time but is of interest. Addis and others attempted to expand the inferences that may be drawn from the appearance of inflammatory cells in the urine. Their operating premise was that the number of pus cells, red cells, or casts shed in the urine per unit of time possesses identifying significance as "to the nature and intensity of the renal lesion" (1). This premise has proved to be disappointing in practice.

It is typical for some renal conditions to cause a greater discharge of inflammatory elements into the urine than others. If two lesions of the kidney were of similar size and location, a richer urinary sediment would likely be observed 1) in an acute versus a chronic process, 2) in a pyogenic versus a granulomatous infection, 3) in an exacerbating versus a quiescent lesion, 4) in an inflammation versus a degeneration, etc. However, these numbers do not provide enough diagnostic correlation to warrant the use of a counting chamber (Addis count). The accuracy of the usual semiquantitative estimation, reported as numbers per microscopic field, is adequate to demonstrate whatever relationship may exist between the number of cells or casts shed and the nature of the renal pathology. Any additional accuracy derived from enumeration in a counting chamber over that of a semiquantitative method is far too little to warrant the time and effort involved. Wells (64) sums up the situation quite appropriately when he states in his book on clinical pathology that, "Most of us find the Addis counts impractical. They yield no more information than ordinary microscopic examinations provided, of course, that the latter are correctly done."

COLLECTION OF SPECIMEN

A 12-hour specimen is used. This is collected in a jug containing 0.5 ml formalin. The patient empties the bladder completely at 7:00 P.M. and discards the urine. All subsequent urine is saved until 7:00 A.M. the next morning, when the bladder is again emptied and this final sample added to the container. On the day of collection, the patient may have breakfast as usual, including fluids, but no further fluids should be taken until the 12-hour urine collection is completed the next morning. Food, on the other hand, is allowed during the collection period.

PROCEDURE

1. Mix the specimen well by repeated inversion, and measure the total amount accurately within 2 ml.
2. With a pipette, transfer 10 ml to a graduated centrifuge tube and centrifuge for 5 min at 1800 RPM. Use a small tabletop centrifuge with low relative centrifugal force (RCF), approximately 500–600.
3. Carefully remove 9 ml supernatant fluid (without stirring up the sediment); using a capillary pipette, thoroughly mix the sediment in the remaining 1 ml volume. If the sediment is heavy, a dilution may be made.
4. Place a sample of the suspended sediment into a Neubauer blood counting chamber as if doing a leukocyte count.
5. The number and differential cast counts are made under low power in all nine large squares (0.0009 ml urine).
6. The RBCs and WBCs are counted in the same area under high power.

CALCULATIONS

The following formula represents the number of cells or casts corrected for a 12-hour time factor and volume:

$$N = \frac{s}{v} \times n \times \frac{V}{10} = \frac{1}{0.0009} \times \text{cells counted} \times \frac{\text{volume}}{10}$$

After the calculations are completed, a report is written on a special laboratory sheet and should include the volume for 12 hours, the number of cells and casts in the 12-hour sample, and a list of the normal values. The normal values for adults are

Casts 0–5,000
RBC 0–500,000
WBC 0–1,000,000

Children may excrete slightly more casts than adults but slightly fewer WBCs and RBCs.

Note. If urates are present, dissolve them by immersing the container in warm water. Also, unless the pH of the urine is 6 or less, some of the casts may have dissolved. This may make certain specimens unsatisfactory for an Addis count. Therefore, the count should be made as soon as possible after receiving the specimen to prevent distortion or destruction of the formed elements.

12 Urinary Pigments

Normally no detectable blood is present in urine; frequently, however, blood may contaminate the urine in menstruating females. Hemoglobin may be present in urine in the form of intact RBCs (hematuria) or as free hemoglobin (hemoglobinuria). Most often some free hemoglobin will accompany RBCs due to lysis of a portion of the cells.

Hematuria may originate from anywhere in the kidneys and urinary tract. Hemoglobinuria may occur from hemolysis of blood circulation and blood excreted by the kidney (as in hemolytic anemias or paroxysmal hemoglobinuria), or it may occur in the urine specimen itself because highly alkaline pH or dilute urines will cause red cells to lyse. This process is further exaggerated if the urine stands for a long time before testing.

Chemical dipstick tests which can detect RBCs as well as hemoglobin are much more sensitive to free hemoglobin. Microscopic examination is necessary to distinguish hematuria from hemoglobinuria. The dipstick will also react with the muscle pigment myoglobin which may be released in muscle injury; however, hemoglobinuria and myoglobinuria are indistinguishable by the benzidine or dipstick test.

MYOGLOBIN

Myoglobin does not originate in the kidney but rather appears in the urine because it is filtered out of the plasma at the glomerulus. Its molecular weight is relatively low (22,000 daltons), and virtually no binding to plasma protein occurs.

Myoglobin originates from breakdown of muscle cells. While breakdown of any muscle cell will result in the release of myoglobin, only the breakdown of skeletal muscle (as distinguished from smooth muscle and myocardium) will result in sufficient myoglobin release to cause pigmenturia.

METHOD

Qualitative determinations for the detection of hemoglobin and myoglobin are routinely done with dipsticks. The reagent area contains peroxide and orthotoluidine. Hemoglobin and myoglobin in urine will catalyze the oxidation of the chromogen orthotoluidine by peroxide. The test is read for blue color at 30 sec and reported as negative to 4+. As little as 0.3 mg/dl is detectable.

INTERFERENCES AND FALSE RESULTS

Sensitivity is reduced by high concentrations of ascorbic acid. In addition, some oxidizing contaminants, *e.g.*, hypochlorite or microbial peroxidase, may cause false-positive reactions.

HEMOGLOBINURIA

The occurrence of erythrocytes in the urine is designated as hematuria (see Erythrocytes, Ch. 5). These red cells may disintegrate and discharge their hemoglobin into the urine; technically this does constitute hemoglobinuria. Hemoglobinuria in the absence of RBCs in the microscopic examination indicates a preceding and causative hemoglobinemia of a sufficient degree to exceed plasma protein binding for hemoglobin, which is approximately 150 mg/dl. Hemoglobinemia of this extent occurs in many conditions: extensive burns; the hemolytic action of certain bacteria, parasites, drugs, and snake venoms; incompatible transfusions; prosthetic heart valves; as well as the crises of such hemolytic diseases as sickle cell anemia, congenital hemolytic anemias, and paroxysmal hemoglobinemias.

If the intravascular hemolytic activity is sufficiently great and thus exceeds the binding capacity of a haptoglobin (a serum protein), the quantity of hemoglobin appearing in the urine is grossly visible. If the pH is low, the color of such urine is dark brown or smoky; but it may be pink if an alkaline reaction exists. Lesser degrees of hemoglobinuria may be detected by the benzidine test.

BENZIDINE OR ORTHOTOLUIDINE TEST FOR BLOOD

To two volumes of urine, add one volume of a saturated solution of benzidine base in glacial acetic acid and one volume of hydrogen peroxide 3%; a resultant blue color indicates hemoglobin. This blue color develops when the benzidine is oxidized, which occurs when oxygen is released from the hydrogen peroxide by the peroxidase activity of hemoglobin or myoglobin. Any other urinary substance, e.g., puss cells, formalin, bromides, iodides, fat, acids, etc., that possesses peroxidaselike activity produces a false-positive test. A false-negative test arises most frequently through the use of defective reagents, faulty proportions of reagents, or the presence of ascorbic acid in large quantities.

Benzidine and orthotoluidine have been for many years the most commonly used chromogens for determination of occult blood in feces. These compounds are now considered carcinogenic, and their continued use for routine analysis has been discouraged. Diphenylamine can replace them. Other substances which have been used in tests for occult blood include phenolphthalein (formed from phenol and phthalic anhydride by boiling an alkaline solution of the indicator with zinc dust), *p*-phenylenediamine chlorhydrate, aminopyrine (amidopyrine, Pyramidon), 3-aminophthalic acid hydrazide, and leucomalachite green (30).

HEMOLYTIC INFECTIONS AND HEMOGLOBINURIA

Occasionally, a specimen is received on an emergency basis from a very ill patient who is obviously feverish, often near coma, and whose urine looks peculiar. On receipt in the laboratory, the urine may be cloudy and rather discolored with a reddish tint. The technologist receiving the specimen should immediately take note of the color and proceed with an examination to demonstrate the nature of the color abnormality.

High fever and systemic infection with hemolytic bacterial microorganisms may result in massive hemolysis with passage of hemoglobin into the urine and extreme damage to renal tubular cells and associated proteinuria. Recognition of this abnormality should be telephoned immediately to the physician in charge. For example, a diabetic patient has been operated on routinely for an acutely inflamed gallbladder. The diagnosis of chronic cholecystitis had been made by the pathologist; but one day later the individual is much more ill, is running a high fever, and shows discolored urine, often with reddish tinge and a protein precipitate. This emergency should be recognized as *life-threatening* and immediately called to the physician's attention as massive hemolysis with hemoglobinuria from a presumed clostridial infection. *Clostridium perfringens* is the organism most commonly involved in such cases because it produces massive necrosis through its lethal necrotizing and hemolytic alpha toxin. The theta toxin of *C. perfringens* is also hemolytic and necrotizing, but it does not hydrolyze lecithin as does the alpha toxin.

HEMOSIDERIN (ROUS TEST)

Hemosiderin, derived from the iron of the hemoglobin molecule, is a dark yellow pigment which may be deposited in the tissues of the body as the result of chronic blood hemolysis such as in hemolytic anemias, pernicious anemia, or sickle cell anemia. In hemochromatosis and hemosiderosis of the kidney, cells containing this pigment may be excreted in the urine. Many free hemosiderin granules may also be excreted. Rous test employs the Prussian blue reaction for iron detection (53).

The reagents are prepared as follows:

1. A 2% solution of potassium ferrocyanide (fresh), prepared by dissolving 1 g potassium ferrocyanide in 50 ml water.
2. A 1% solution of HCl, prepared by mixing 2 ml HCl 5% and 8 ml distilled water.

Rous test is performed as follows:

1. Centrifuge a fresh sample of urine in the usual manner.
2. Pour off the supernatant urine. (The sediment may be examined for brown granules indicating hemosiderin.)
3. Make a mixture of 5 ml potassium ferrocyanide 2% and 5 ml of HCl 1%, and suspend the rest of the sediment in this mixture.
4. Allow the mixture to stand for 10 min. Centrifuge the mixture and examine microscopically for granules of hemosiderin which will appear blue. A coverslip will aid in the microscopic examination.

BILIRUBIN (BILE)

Hemoglobin consists of a complex of four heme molecules, each composed of protoporphyrin and iron, linked to a protein (globin). When erythrocytes are destroyed and hemoglobin degraded by the reticuloendothelial system, the protein is split off for reutilization in the nitrogen pool; the iron is returned to the iron pool for hemoglobin resynthesis, leaving the porphyrin ring fraction. The porphyrin ring fraction is then broken and by a series of reactions transformed into the pigment bilirubin.

Bilirubin is then carried from these cells to the liver cells by an albumin molecule (unconjugated bilirubin or verdohemoglobin). When the bilirubin reaches the liver, the albumin is released. Through the action of the enzyme glucuronyl transferase, bilirubin is conjugated with glucuronic acid (2).

The conjugated bilirubin is then secreted into the bile duct and is excreted into the intestine where it is converted to urobilinogen. In liver diseases, in which there is cell necrosis or obstruction of the bile ducts, the bilirubin cannot be excreted into the intestine; this block results in spilling over of these substances into the bloodstream and excretion in the urine.

BILIRUBINURIA

Bilirubin diglucuronide at low levels in the blood is readily filtered at the glomerulus and promptly appears in the urine. Unconjugated bilirubin (verdohemoglobin) is bound to albumin and as a consequence cannot pass through the glomerular capillary membrane even though it may accumulate to a high blood concentration.

The normal blood level of conjugated bilirubin is less than 0.1 mg/dl, while that of the unconjugated variety ranges 0.5–0.8 mg/dl. Neither of these concentrations is sufficient to result in a positive test for bilirubinuria. Verdohemoglobin levels of the blood may be increased severalfold without producing bilirubinuria, but a level of 1 or 2 mg conjugated bilirubin (the direct-acting van den Bergh pigment complex) per 100 ml of blood produces bilirubinuria.

There are many different methods for detecting bilirubinuria. Bile imparts a yellow brown color to urine; and due to its influence on surface tension, the foam of agitated urine is yellow if bile is present.

HARRISON SPOT TEST

One of the better tests for bilirubin detection, because of its simplicity, is the Harrison spot test. This is performed as follows:

1. Impregnate filter paper strips with a saturated solution of barium chloride and then allow them to dry.
2. Moisten the strip with Fouchet's reagent (trichloroacetic acid 25% in aqueous ferric chloride 1% solution) and then add two to three drops of urine.
3. Various shades of blue and green indicate a positive test.

DIPSTICK

A diazo compound derived from 2,4-dinitroaniline, when coupled with urine bilirubin in a strong acid medium, gives a tan or brown color within 20 sec. This reagent area is found on Bili-labstix and Multistix (see Table

6–1) which are very convenient for routine analysis, but this method is less sensitive than the Ictotest (Ames Company). Urines giving questionable color reactions or those suspected of containing very small amounts of bilirubin should be tested with Ictotest.

ICTOTEST

Five drops of urine are placed on a small square of test mat. One Ictotest tablet (containing p-nitrobenzene-diazonium-p-toluenesulfonate, sulfosalicylic acid, sodium bicarbonate, and boric acid) is placed on the urine, and two drops of distilled water are placed on the tablet to dissolve the reagents. The area about the base of the tablet is observed for the development of a blue or purple color on the mat within 30 sec. The test is negative if no blue or purple color develops on the mat within 30 sec. Results are usually reported as either positive (weak or strong) or negative. This method is four to eight times more sensitive than the dipstick test.

INTERFERENCES AND FALSE RESULTS

Color reactions which might be mistaken for positive bilirubin (on the dipstick) occur with patients receiving large doses of chlorpromazine. Metabolites of Pyridium and ethoxazene hydrochloride (Serenium) may give red or other color to the test area, but these are usually not confused with positive brown colors.

UROBILINOGEN

Urobilinogen refers to a group of pigmented compounds normally present in the stool and in the urine in small amounts. An increase in urine urobilinogen, as well as the presence of urine bilirubin, is one of the first indications of liver disorder. Frequently urine urobilinogen and bilirubin determinations are valuable in distinguishing biliary obstruction from hepatic disorders in jaundiced patients.

UROBILINOGENURIA AND UROBILINURIA

A complete discussion of hemoglobin pigment metabolism would be out of place in a discussion of urinalysis. However, it is necessary to present a partial outline of pigment degradation and disposition in order to evaluate the significance of several tests that frequently are performed upon urine.

The liver parenchyma converts the verdohemoglobin of lysed red cells (also known as unconjugated bilirubin or the indirect-acting van den

Bergh pigment complex) to conjugated bilirubin and excretes it via the common bile duct into the small intestine as a component of bile. Intestinal bacteria reduce this conjugated bilirubin mainly by oxygenation into a group of closely related, colorless substances known collectively as urobilinogens. Urobilinogen, when oxidized to brownish urobilin by contact with oxygen from the air, imparts the familiar brown color to feces.

Small quantities of urobilinogen are reabsorbed from the intestinal tract and are returned to the liver where the urobilinogen is extracted and reexcreted in the bile, probably after reconversion to bilirubin. However, a small percentage of the urobilinogen reabsorbed from the intestine escapes the liver and goes into the general circulation. The kidneys handle this blood urobilinogen as though it were a foreign substance, *i.e.*, the tubular cells do not actively reabsorb the filtered urobilinogen. Consequently urobilinogenuria is a normal occurrence. The quantity of urobilinogen that the average adult excretes daily in urine ranges from a trace to 4 mg; the latter represents an amount sufficient to give a qualitatively positive test with the urine diluted up to 20 times.

The amount of urinary urobilinogen is directly related to the rate of red cell breakdown if other processes are normal. Increased urinary urobilinogen is found in hemolytic episodes but also may be observed in the absence of excessive hemolysis if an ailing liver permits a greater percentage of the portally returned urobilinogen to escape into the general circulation.

On the other hand, if bile fails to reach the intestinal tract for conversion, the urinary urobilinogen level falls to zero regardless of the rate of red cell destruction or the functional status of the liver parenchyma. Stones, tumors, or other causes of obstruction to biliary outflow prevent formation of urobilinogen in the intestines.

Urobilin is the colored oxidation product of urobilinogen, and both have the same significance in urine. The test for urobilin is more difficult and less precise than the test for urobilinogen. It is common practice to use fresh urine and to test for urobilinogen before contact with the air converts it to urobilin.

METHODS FOR DETECTION OF UROBILINOGEN

To 10 ml urine, add 1 ml Ehrlich's benzaldehyde reagent. A pink to cherry red color developing in 10 min indicates urobilinogen is present. For practical purposes quantitation is best done by the dilution method. Ehrlich's reagent also reacts with porphobilinogen.

Dipstick Method

Some dipsticks contain a test area for urobilinogen which contains *p*-dimethylaminobenzaldehyde. The color reaction is read after exactly 60 sec. The number of units (Ehrlich units) and the normal range (0.1–1 Ehrlich units) are reported.

Interferences and False Results

Pyridium and azo dyes in a urine specimen may give the appearance of an elevated urobilinogen or may mask the true color development. In such cases the dipstick method is not reliable. False-positive reactions may be seen with Ehrlich-reacting substances such as porphobilinogen or *p*-aminosalicylic acid.

PORPHOBILINOGEN AND PORPHYRINS

Porphyrins and porphobilinogen are important intermediate compounds in the pathway to protoporphyrin formation. As such, they are precursors of the hemoglobins and cytochromes. The major production sites of these substances are the liver and bone marrow. Protoporphyrin synthesis begins with glycine and succinate, which are combined to form δ aminolevulinic acid (δ ALA). Porphobilinogen, composed of a single pyrrole ring, is subsequently formed. Four of these rings are joined with various side chains, resulting in the porphyrin compounds (coproporphyrin and uroporphyrin). These porphyrins precede protoporphyrin and heme. Normally there are very small amounts of coproporphyrins, uroporphyrins, and porphobilinogen in urine and feces.

Porphobilinogen is a colorless compound but converts to red porphobilin and uroporphyrin after excretion. Normal urinary excretion is up to 2 mg/day. Porphyrins may exist in the body as two isomers, types I and III. Under abnormal situations uroporphyrin I and coproporphyrin I are formed. The normal pathway produces coproporphyrin and uroporphyrin III. Normal urinary excretion of coproporphyrin is about 30–180 μg/day; of uroporphyrin, about 10–30 μg/day. Elevated quantities of porphyrins are known to give urine a port wine color.

Except for trace amounts of coproporphyrin, porphyrins are not formed during the normal physiologic degradation of hemoglobin. Instead, the cyclic configuration of the porphyrins is lost by cleavage of the alpha methene bridge of hemoglobin's protoporphyrin, thereby creating the straight chain complex known as bilirubin (unconjugated bilirubin). Conjugation in the liver with glucuronic acid, followed by further reductions and oxidations in the intestine, result in the formation of urobilinogens and urobilins, respectively.

Porphyrins are named according to the nature of the side chains that are substituted onto the eight available positions on the four pyrrole complexes of the porphyrin nucleus (Fig. 12–1):

Protoporphyrin: Four methyl, two proprionyl, and two vinyl groups
Coproporphyrin: Four methyl and four proprionic acid groups
Uroporphyrin: Four acetic acid and four proprionic acid groups

Coproporphyrins (isomers I and III) are excreted daily in amounts that total 50–100 μg in the urine and 150–400 μg in the feces. Normally, neither porphobilinogen nor uroporphyrin is excreted in detectable amounts in either feces or urine.

Porphyrinuria indicates excessive urinary excretion of any type of porphyrin and the presence of porphobilinogen in the urine. In the porphyrinurias due to uroporphyrins, the urine is usually brown red when voided; it darkens on exposure to sunlight, even if there is no redness when the urine is voided. Also, urine specimens containing large quantities of porphobilinogen, as in the acquired porphyrias, may be red brown when voided or may develop this color upon standing because the colorless

Fig. 12–1. Naming of porphyrins.

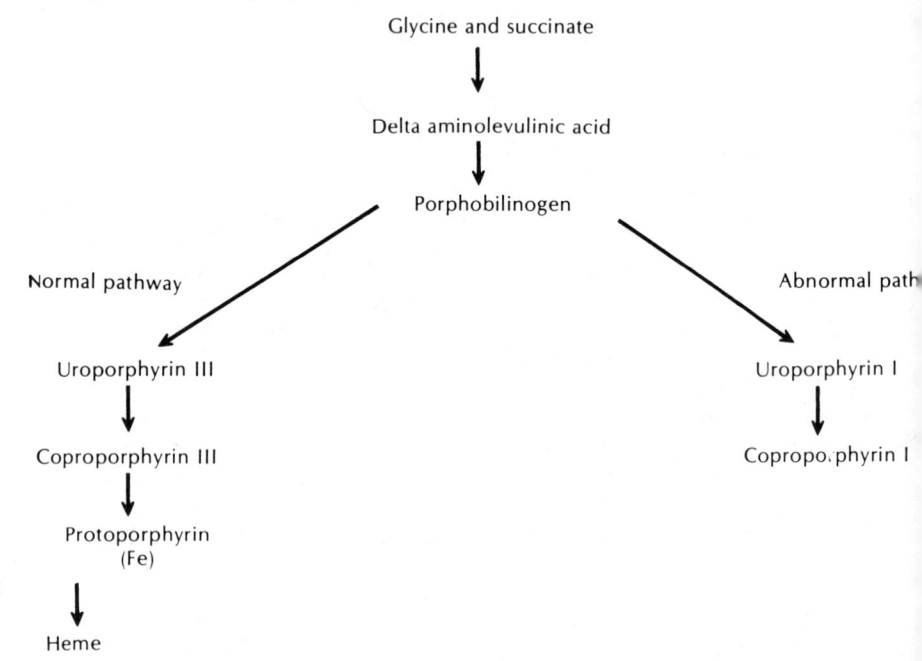

Glycine and succinate
↓
Delta aminolevulinic acid
↓
Porphobilinogen

Normal pathway / Abnormal path

Uroporphyrin III → Uroporphyrin I
↓ ↓
Coproporphyrin III Copropo.phyrin I
↓
Protoporphyrin (Fe)
↓
Heme

porphobilinogen changes into either one or both of two red substances, *i.e.*, uroporphyrin or porphobilin.

The physical signs and laboratory findings in the porphyrinurias can better be appreciated by a review of some of the properties of porphyrins.

1. Coproporphyrins and especially uroporphyrins exhibit fluorescence when viewed in the ultraviolet light. Porphobilinogen does not exhibit fluorescence.
2. Urine specimens that contain uroporphyrins (and coproporphyrins) are dark red. Exposure to sunlight increases the intensity of the color and may make weak concentrations of urinary porphyrins apparent.
3. Alkaline urine samples that contain only porphobilinogen are colorless in reaction. Exposure to sunlight does not alter the color appreciably if the urine remains alkaline. Acidifying the sample containing porphobilinogen results in a color change which is intensified by exposure to light with the passage of time (uroporphyrin and porphobilin are formed).
4. The Watson–Schwartz test is negative with both porphobilin and porphyrins but is positive with porphobilinogen (and urobilinogen).
5. Uroporphyrins are deposited in teeth, bones, and skin, and with their eight active carboxyl radicals are sufficiently reactive with light to produce a severe dermal reaction on slight sunlight exposure. Neither coproporphyrins nor porphobilinogen is similarly reactive to sunlight.

Porphyria refers to a group of clinical disorders in which porphyrin (and occasionally porphobilinogen) production is increased. Such conditions are due to genetic or metabolic disorders in which the abnormalities are in the synthesis of the compounds. They may be congenital or acquired. Porphyrinuria refers to the presence of elevated quantities of porphyrins, especially of coproporphyrin, excreted in the urine. The abnormality does not lie with the metabolic process but rather is secondary to another condition.

ERYTHROPOIETIC PORPHYRIA

Erythropoietic porphyria, inherited as a recessive congenital disorder, is probably the most severe porphyria. Due to deficient or defective enzymes, large amounts of uroporphyrin I and coproporphyrin I are produced by the bone marrow, deposited in subcutaneous tissues and organs, and excreted in urine. Porphobilinogen is not increased. Symptoms, which are noticeable in childhood, include skin eruptions, photosensitivity, and anemia. Urine is usually pink or burgundy.

A number of conditions may be responsible for porphyrinuria. These include liver cirrhosis, anemias, chemical poisoning, some drugs, febrile states, biliary obstruction, and hepatitis. Also some infections, rheumatic fever, infectious mononucleosis, and some cases of pellagra can produce porphyrinuria.

With the congenital type, the urinary findings include:

1. Color: deep red, increasing on exposure to sunlight
2. Pigment: large quantities of uroporphyrin I, smaller quantities of coproporphyrin I and III, no porphobilinogen
3. Tests: positive ultraviolet fluorescence test, positive spectroscopic test for uroporphyrin, ether-insoluble property of uroporphyrin, negative Watson–Schwartz test.

ACUTE, INTERMITTENT PORPHYRIA

With the acquired (acute), intermittent type of porphyria, the metabolic derangement is characterized by the production and excretion of large quantities of porphobilinogen. Porphobilinogen, a complex pyrrole, is a colorless compound that does not fluoresce in ultraviolet light. Consequently there is no discoloration or fluorescence of teeth or other tissues and similarly no light sensitivity of the skin. Nevertheless, the urine may be red brown when voided and deepens in color upon standing. As previously explained, this is due to the formation in an acid medium of uroporphyrin and porphobilin from the porphobilinogen. Symptoms include intermittent acute abdominal pain, neurologic disorders, and possibly skin eruptions. Certain drugs, *e.g.*, barbiturates and alcohol, may precipitate an attack. The urinary findings include:

1. Color: normal yellow, may be red or may become red brown on standing if acidic
2. Pigment: colorless chromogen (porphobilinogen) initially; may develop uroporphyrins and porphobilin from the porphobilinogen
3. Tests: positive Watson–Schwartz test for porphobilinogen; may develop positive tests for uroporphyrins on standing

PORPHYRIA CUTANEA TARDA

Porphyria cutanea tarda resembles porphyria erythropoietica clinically, with features of acute intermittent porphyria, and also causes porphyrinuria. The onset occurs later in life and is due to a defect in liver metabolism. Elevated urinary porphyrins and δ ALA are present, but porphobilinogen is only rarely increased. Symptoms include photosensitivity and many skin eruptions. The urine is usually red. Acquired porphyria cutanea tarda is an occasional complication of alcoholic cirrhosis.

COPROPORPHYRINS

Coproporphyrins (isomers I and III) appear in the urine in a large variety of disease states and seem to indicate a less severe derangement of pyrrole metabolism than does either uroporphyrinuria or porphobilinogenuria. In fact, the coproporphyrins, even when produced in large quantities, do not appear to contribute to the symptomatology of the disease entities in which they are found.

Because coproporphyrins possess a relatively weak fluorescent quality and impart color to urine, they require differentiation from the uroporphyrins. They may be recognized by the spectroscope as well as by the fact that they are soluble in acetic acid–ether mixture, while uroporphyrins are insoluble in this reagent.

Large amounts of coproporphyrin (isomer I) have been excreted in the urine in the presence of intoxication by lead, mercury, and other heavy metals.

Coproporphyrin (isomer III) has been reported to be excreted in large amounts in the urine in conditions with a neuropathic component, *e.g.*, poliomyelitis, aplastic anemia, chronic alcoholism, and especially lead poisoning which is characteristically associated with elevated urinary coproporphyrin III and δ ALA. Lead inhibits the conversion of δ ALA to porphobilinogen, coproporphyrin III to protoporphyrin, and the incorporation of iron into protoporphyrin.

WATSON–SCHWARTZ TEST

The Watson–Schwartz test (63) is used to detect porphobilinogen and is not positive with either porphobilin or the porphyrins. Since porphobilinogen changes in an acidic medium to porphobilin and/or uroporphyrin, the test must be made promptly with freshly voided urine.

The porphobilinogen screen is carried out as follows:

1. In a test tube mix 2 ml urine and 2 ml modified Ehrlich's reagent (0.7 grams *p*-dimethylaminobenzaldehyde, 150 ml concentrated HCl, and 100 ml distilled water).
2. Add 4 ml saturated sodium acetate (zinc acetate may be used) buffer and mix. The development of a pink color after step 1 or step 2 indicates reaction of Ehrlich's reagent with urinary substances, but this reaction is not specific for porphobilinogen.
3. Add a few ml chloroform and *mix well*. Porphobilinogen is *insoluble* in chloroform, while other Ehrlich-reacting compounds, *e.g.*, urobilinogen, are soluble in chloroform.
4. The test reading is based on the presence of color in the aqueous (top) layer. A dark pink color in the aqueous (top) layer with a clear chloro-

form (bottom) layer is positive for porphobilinogen. Absence of this pink color from the aqueous layer, regardless of the color of the chloroform, is negative for porphobilinogen. When a pink color is present in both layers, extraction of the aqueous layer may continue until the pink color is absent from either aqueous or chloroform layers so that the reading can be made clearly.

WATSON'S TEST

As a porphyrin screen, Watson's test is carried out as follows:

1. In a separatory funnel mix 25 ml urine and 10 ml glacial acetic acid.
2. Add 50 ml ether and mix well. The ether (top) layer will contain coproporphyrins while the uroporphyrins are left in the aqueous (bottom) layer.
3. Remove this aqueous (bottom) layer.
4. To the ether layer remaining in the separatory funnel, add 10 ml HCl 5% and mix. The coproporphyrins will be extracted into the HCl (bottom) layer. Remove this layer to a test tube.
5. Under Wood's lamp (ultraviolet light), observe both the aqueous layer from step 3 and the HCl layer from step 4, looking for a pink fluorescence in both cases. A pink fluorescence indicates porphyrins in increased amounts. Report as increased or not increased.

Urinary pigments left in the aqueous layer may interfere by masking the fluorescence of uroporphyrins.

MELANIN

Urine which contains melanin, like urine with homogentisic acid, darkens on exposure to air, assuming a dark brown or black color. Melanin does not reduce copper, however, as do the alkapton bodies. Melanuria occurs to some degree in most cases of metastatic malignant melanoma but may rarely be observed in other diseases. The substance eliminated in the urine is melanogen, a colorless precursor of melanin. On oxidation, as by ferric chloride, melanogen becomes melanin, which is brown black (53).

Procedures for testing for melanin are as follows:

1. Addition of a few drops of a solution of ferric chloride to 10 ml urine gives a gray precipitate which blackens on standing.
2. Bromine water added to urine in equal proportions causes a yellow precipitate which gradually turns black.

Thormählen's test for melanogen is carried out as follows:

1. To 5 ml urine in a test tube, add a few drops of sodium nitroprusside solution; then add a few drops of NaOH 10%.
2. A deep ruby color develops which is not specific for melanogen, since it also indicates acetone and creatinine.
3. Acidify with glacial acetic acid. The immediate development of an azure color indicates the presence of melanogen. With acetone alone, the color becomes deeper red; with creatinine it becomes yellow, then green, and finally blue.

CAROTENE, VITAMIN A, AND RELATED PIGMENTS

A number of naturally occurring pigments called carotenoids are precursors of vitamin A. They range in color from yellow to purple. Beta-carotene is a principal carotenoid in serum and may appear in urine. Normally, carotenoids are in the lipoprotein fraction of serum. They are measured by a process involving hydrolysis of the protein complex, saponification, and extraction with isooctane. One aliquot is transferred to a microcuvette for measurement of carotene content at 450 nm. Another aliquot is evaporated to dryness, following which the residue is dissolved in chloroform and then reacted with dichloropropanol. Vitamin A forms a blue color which changes to violet, and its absorbance is measured at 550 nm (30).

Thiamine, or vitamin B_1, is normally present in free form in serum and in the red cells of blood. An excess of thiamine in the urine occurs usually in a person, often an alcoholic, taking large quantities of the vitamin in an attempt to recover normal liver function. The urine becomes a bright yellowish color slightly different from the usual golden color of the urochrome pigments. Its measurement in body fluids is by an oxidative conversion with ferricyanide and an alkaline solution to a thiochrome. The product is a fluorescent and is extracted for fluorometric measurements (30).

13 Urine Fat

Normally urine does not contain fat; however, fat may be found in the urine with some conditions. For example, fat may find its way into urine after crushing injuries to the long bones. In patients with multiple fractures, fat may be released from bone marrow, circulated, and passed through the glomerular membrane. Urine fat is significant as an indication that fat droplets have been released into the bloodstream where they may form emboli and cause infarction. Fat may also appear in the urine as a result of nephritis or may arise from degenerating epithelial cells from the urinary tract.

The presence of fat in renal cystic fluid and a variety of other fluids of the body may also be of interest. A simple qualitative test for fat employs the fat-soluble Sudan stain. This procedure is performed as follows:

1. To approximately 10 ml urine or fluid in a conical centrifuge tube, add several drops of Sudan stain.
2. Mix well and allow to stand for 1–2 min.
3. Skim the top of the fluid to obtain Sudan-stained fat droplets for microscopic study.
4. Centrifuge for 4 min (as for a routine microscopic sediment examination).
5. Remove supernatant fluid and mix sediment well. Coverslip a drop of sediment and examine microscopically for red or golden-colored, round, glistening bodies.
6. Report a number range of fat globules per high-power field.

Fat is revealed with striking clarity when the light transmitted through the urine is polarized. In this situation, the fat (whether free floating or within cells) appears as brilliantly refractile bodies with the Maltese cross pattern.

14 Calcium

The amount of calcium in the urine is the difference between what is filtered at the glomerulus and what is subsequently reabsorbed by the tubular system of the kidney. Although not true of some substances (such as glucose, sodium, etc.), the entire measured concentration of serum calcium is unavailable for filtration at the glomerulus. This is because about half of the measured serum calcium is bound to albumin; just as albumin itself cannot pass through the glomerulus, neither can the calcium bound to the albumin pass through. The unbound calcium (almost exclusively ionized) is the fraction of the serum calcium which imparts physiologic effects and is subject to physiologic control.

For example, if we presume that unbound (ionized) calcium concentration is 4.5 mg/dl with a measured plasma concentration of 9 mg/dl and that the glomerular filtration rate is 100 ml/min, then the amount of calcium filtered per minute is the product of plasma ionized calcium concentration times glomerular filtration rate. In this case, 4.5 mg/dl multiplied by 100 ml/min would yield a product of 4.5 mg/min, which is the amount of calcium filtered per minute. If this product is then multiplied by 1440 (the number of minutes per day), one would obtain the number of mg calcium filtered per day:

$$4.5 \times 1440 = 6480 \text{ mg/day}$$

The urine of a normal individual on a normal diet contains less than 250 mg/day of calcium. Therefore, continuing with our example, 6480 mg/day less 250 mg/day (normal) would equal 6230 mg/day; or, at a maximum, approximately 4% of the calcium filtered at the glomerulus appears in the urine, indicating that at least 96% of the filtered calcium is reabsorbed.

The amount of calcium appearing in the urine is related to the quantity filtered at the glomerulus (a product of glomerular filtration rate and the ionized plasma calcium concentration) and the quantity reabsorbed. As a consequence, the concentration of calcium in the urine is a relatively poor indicator of the plasma concentration. In addition, the absolute concentration of calcium in the urine is controlled by factors which may be quite unrelated to calcium excretion, *i.e.*, the concentration of the urine.

METHOD

One of the most accurate methods for measuring the concentration of calcium in the urine utilizes the principles of atomic absorption spectroscopy. With appropriate dilutions, the automated chemical analyzer will also yield a reasonably accurate measurement of urine calcium. In either form of measurement, the proper collection of the specimen is of critical importance. Most calcium salts become less soluble as the urine pH increases. If urine stands and bacteriologic degradation of urea to ammonia occurs, the excreted calcium largely precipitates out of solution and is not measured. This problem is easily avoided by adding a few drops of concentrated hydrochloric acid to the collection container. This maneuver sufficiently acidifies the urine to prevent precipitation.

A much less sensitive test for urine calcium is the Sulkowitch test. This test is rapid but imprecise. A normal individual's urine has 1+ to 2+ flocculation. A negative test suggests that the ionized concentration of calcium is quite low in the plasma or that the glomerular filtration rate is sharply reduced. A 3+ to 4+ flocculation suggests excessive calcium excretion and perhaps increased plasma concentration of calcium. However, this latter interpretation may be erroneous if calcium reabsorption has been impaired. The Sulkowitch test is performed with a reagent made of oxalic acid, 2.5 g; ammonium oxalate, 2.5 g; glacial acetic acid, 5 ml; and distilled water q.s., 150 ml. To approximately 10 parts of the supernatant of centrifuged urine is added one part of the Sulkowitch reagent and the solution is mixed. The subsequent degree of turbidity is estimated by a scale of 0 (no precipitate) to 4+ or positive (a flocculent precipitate). This precipitate is calcium oxalate. The report may be stated to be negative (containing no precipitate), trace to 2+ or normal (light precipitate or fine, white cloudy precipitate), 3+ to 4+ or positive (heavy, milklike or very heavy, cloudy precipitate).

RENAL CALCULUS ANALYSIS

Stone (calculus) analysis for chemical constituents is a difficult procedure. Several regional laboratories exist for performing this type of analysis.

15 Generalized Metabolic Derangements

INBORN ERRORS OF METABOLISM

In 1923 Garrod (27) listed only six conditions due to inborn errors of metabolism: albinism, cystinuria, alkaptonuria, porphyrinuria, steatorrhea, and pentosuria. Throughout the years many other conditions have been added to this list of inheritable metabolic derangements. However, the concern here is with only a few of the conditions which may be detected by urinary examination.

In 1965 Efron (23) classified aminoacidurias as 1) inherited secondary aminoaciduria, 2) primary overflow aminoaciduria, 3) no-threshold aminoaciduria, and 4) renal transport aminoaciduria. The best recent review of this subject matter can be found in the book by Thomas and Howell (61) published in 1973 entitled *Selected Screening Tests for Genetic Metabolic Diseases* (Tables 15–1 through 15–5).

SCREENING TESTS

Screening is usually defined as the application of a medical test to large numbers of individuals volunteering to be tested because of a probable health benefit. The aim of genetic screening is to find individuals with a potentially fatal or debilitating genetic disease or individuals with a genetic predisposition to acute or chronic illness for which there is an ameliorative treatment. Screening may also be designed to detect persons with a high probability of producing genetically damaged children. Such persons identified are most often heterozygous carriers of a defect that will lead to genetic disease in a proportion of their offspring. In the past only a tragic index case provided the first indication of hereditary disease when both parents were carriers.

Screening procedures should be reliable and reproducible, sensitive and specific; that is, there must be a low number of false-positive and false-negative tests. Screening distinguishes the abnormal from the normal but may not clearly distinguish between phenotypes resulting from genetic heterogeneity. For this reason, confirming tests are an essential component of genetic screening.

Preliminary screening tests are usually simple, inexpensive, and utilize readily available specimens such as blood or urine; confirming tests are likely to be more complex and sophisticated and more expensive. They may utilize less readily available specimens such as tissues, skin fibroblast cultures and saliva, amniotic fluid and cells or tears (51).

TABLE 15-1. INHERITED DISORDERS OF AMINO ACID METABOLISM ASSOCIATED WITH A LOW RENAL CLEARANCE (HIGH THRESHOLD) OF THE AFFECTED AMINO ACID

Disorder	Amino acid(s) increased in blood and urine
Alaninemia	Alanine
Argininemia	Arginine*
Citrullinemia	Citrulline
Glycinemia, nonketotic	Glycine
Glycinemia, ketotic†	Glycine
Histidinemia	Histidine
Hydroxyprolinemia	Hydroxyproline
Hyperammonemia, type I	Glycine and glutamine
Hyperammonemia, type II	Glutamine
Lysinemia, persistent	Lysine
Lysinemia, associated with hyperammonemia	Lysine and arginine
Maple syrup urine disease	Alloisoleucine, isoleucine, leucine, and valine
Methioninemia	Methionine
Oasthouse disease‡	Isoleucine, leucine methionine, pheynlalanine and tyrosine
Ornithinemia	Ornithine
Phenylketonuria and its variants	Phenylalanine
Pipecolatemia	Pipecolic acid
Prolinemia, type I	Proline§
Prolinemia, type II	Proline§
Sarcosinemia	Sarcosine
Tryptophanuria	Tryptophan
Tyrosinemia	Tyrosine¶
Valinemia	Valine

*Arginine, cystine, lysine and ornithine found in urine.

†May be due to a number of different specific defects including propionyl CoA carboxylase deficiency and methylmalonic aciduria.

‡It has been suggested that the oasthouse disease may be identical to the methionine malabsorption syndrome. If this suggestion is confirmed this disorder may be more properly considered an inherited disorder of amino acid transport.

§Proline, hydroxyproline, and glycine increased in urine.

¶Generalized increase in amino acids often found in urine.

(Thomas GH, Howell RR: Selected Screening Tests for Genetic Metabolic Diseases. Chicago, Year Book Medical, 1973)

TABLE 15-2. NONINHERITED CONDITIONS ASSOCIATED WITH CHANGES IN SERUM AMINO ACIDS

Condition	Amino acid changes
Transient tyrosinemia of premature infants	Tyrosine
Neonatal hypermethioninemia	Hyperaminoacidemia, methionine most prominent
Neonatal hyperhydroxyprolinemia	Hydroxyproline
Neonatal hyperphenylalaninemia	Phenylalanine*
Liver necrosis	Hyperaminoacidemia, tyrosine, and methionine most prominent
Certain infections	Varies with disease and stage of disorder

*Often occurs with tyrosinemia.
(Thomas GH, Howell RR: Selected Screening Tests for Genetic Metabolic Diseases. Chicago, Year Book Medical, 1973)

TABLE 15-3. INHERITED DISORDERS OF AMINO ACID METABOLISM ASSOCIATED WITH A HIGH RENAL CLEARANCE (LOW THRESHOLD) OF THE AFFECTED AMINO ACID

Disorder	Amino acids increased in urine
β-Alaninemia	β-Aminoisobutyric acid, γ-aminobutyric acid and taurine
β-Aminoisobutyric aciduria	β-Aminoisobutytic acid
Argininosuccinic aciduria	Argininosuccinic acid and citrulline
Aspartylglycosaminuria	Aspartylglycosamine
Carnosinemia	Carnosine
Cystathionuria	Cystathionine
Homocystinuria	Homocystine
Hypophosphatasia	Phosphoethanolamine
Imidazole amino aciduria	Carnosine, anserine, homocarnosine and methylhistidine
β-Mercaptolactate-cysteine disulfiduria	Mercaptolactate-cysteine disulfide
Sulfite oxidase deficiency	Sulfocysteine

(Thomas GH, Howell RR: Selected Screening for Genetic Metabolic Diseases. Chicago, Year Book Medical, 1973)

TABLE 15-4. INHERITED DISORDERS OF AMINO ACID TRANSPORT

Disorder	Amino Acids Increased in Urine
Cystinuria, types I, II, III	Arginine, cystine, lysine and ornithine
Dibasic aminoaciduria	Arginine, lysine and ornithine
Hartnup disease	Neutral aminoaciduria (except imino acids and glycine)
Hypercystinuria	Cystine
Iminoglycinuria	Glycine, hydroxyproline and proline
Luder-Sheldon syndrome	Generalized aminoaciduria
Methionine malabsorption	Methionine, smaller amounts of tyrosine, phenylalanine, valine and leucine
Glucoglycinuria	Glycine
Glycinuria with hypophosphatemia	Glycine
Glycinuria*	Glycine
Familial protein intolerance	Lysine, also sometimes arginine

*May reflect the heterozygous phenotype of the iminoglycinuric disorder (Thomas GH, Howell RR: Selected Screening Tests for Genetic Metabolic Diseases. Chicago, Year Book Medical, 1973)

TABLE 15-5. INHERITED DISORDERS ASSOCIATED WITH SECONDARY AMINOACIDURIAS PRESUMABLY DUE TO PROGRESSIVE IMPAIRMENT OF RENAL TUBULES

Disorder	Amino acids increased in urine
"Busby" syndrome	Generalized aminoaciduria
Cystinosis	Generalized aminoaciduria
Fanconi syndrome (idiopathic)	Generalized aminoaciduria
Fructose intolerance	Generalized aminoaciduria
Galactosemia	Generalized aminoaciduria
Glycogen storage disease, type I (rarely)	Generalized aminoaciduria
Lactose intolerance	Generalized aminoaciduria
Lowe's syndrome	Generalized aminoaciduria
Tyrosinosis	Generalized aminoaciduria
Wilson's disease	Generalized aminoaciduria

(Thomas GH, Howell RR: Selected Screening Tests for Genetic Metabolic Diseases. Chicago, Year Book Medical, 1973)

A useful starting screen consists of the ferric chloride test, the dinitrophenolhydrazine (DNPH) tests and the nitroprusside test. Bradley (10) indicates the positive and negative findings in the common aminoacidurias (Table 15–6). The reagents for these tests are shown in Table 15–7.

Berry et al. (8) proposed a scheme for detection of metabolic disorders using commercial dip tests, spot plate tests, and chromatographic tests. Bindel (9) described a method utilizing a gas chromatograph/mass spectrometer/computer system.

For chromatography, no pretreatment of the urine specimen is advocated other than thymol and refrigeration. One-dimensional chromatograms can be prepared with urine spots 3 cm apart. Each amino acid can be identified by its characteristic position on the chromatogram. To make quantitative measurements, chromatograms of known amounts of standard amino acids are prepared and run for quality and quantification controls. Two-dimensional chromatograms of amino acids are exceptionally useful in separating them. Spot plate tests, dip tests, and one-dimensional chromatograms can be used to confirm that the urine tested is normal or is not normal.

INITIAL SCREENING

In regard to screening, Berry et al. (8) state:

Each urine specimen is tested with spot tests and commercial dip sticks. Test strips of Combistix* for pH, protein, and glucose, and Phenistix* for phenylpyruvic acid or aspirin, are dipped in the urine. Ketostix,* showing the presence of ketones, and Galatest,† indicating the presence of reducing sugars, are used as described by the manufacturers. The urine is also tested with Millon's reagent for tyrosine and parahydroxyphenyl compounds; with 2,4-dinitrophenylhydrazine for keto acids; and with anthrone reagents to show the presence of all carbohydrates, including nonreducing sugars. Cyanide–nitroprusside reagent is used to detect cystine and homocystine.

Table 15–8 describes the preparation of reagents.

SPOT PLATE AND DIP TESTS

Sugar spot tests are used for detection of abnormalities in carbohydrate excretion (Table 15–9). Such abnormalities can further be confirmed by chromatography.

Phenistix with phenylpyruvic acid produces a green color; with aspirin, a purple color; with bilirubin, a greenish color. Ketostix is quite sensitive for acetone and also produces a positive reaction with pyruvic acid.

*Ames Company, Elkhart, Ind.
†Denver Chemical Company, Denver, Colo.

TABLE 15-6. URINARY SCREENING TESTS FOR INBORN ERRORS OF METABOLISM: AMINOACIDURIA

Disease	Ferric chloride test	DNPH* test	Nitroprusside-cyanide test
Phenylketonuria	Green	+	−
Homocystinuria	−	−	+
Cystinuria	−	−	+
Maple syrup disease	−	+	−
Histidinemia	Olive	±	−
Tyrosinosis	Quick-fading green	+	−
Hyperlysinemia	−	+	−
Hyperglycinemia	−	+	±

*2,4-dinitrophenylhydrazine.
(Bradley MD: Hum Path 2(2):309–320, 1971)

TABLE 15-7. SPOT PLATE TESTS

Reagent	Preparation of reagent	Test & positive reaction
Anthrone	0.05 g anthrone + 25 ml conc H_2SO_4	3 drops urine + 12 drops anthrone; mix with glass stirring rod. Positive: green to dark blue
2,4-Dinitrophenyl-hydrazine	0.3% (w/v) in 1 N HCl	2 drops urine + 2 drops reagent; let stand 5 min & add 2 drops 10% (w/v) NaOH; stir with glass rod. Positive: reddish brown which persists
Millon's reagent	10 g mercury dissolved in 11 ml conc HNO_3 and then diluted with 22 ml H_2O	2 drops urine + 2 drops reagent. Positive: pink or pink brown
Nitroprusside–cyanide	10% (w/v) sodium cyanide; 1% (w/v) sodium nitro-prusside	5 drops urine + 1 drop sodium cyanide; let stand 1 min; add 1 drop sodium nitroprusside. Positive: immediate red pink (magenta) for cystine or homocystine; purple indicates ketone bodies

(Berry HK, Leonard C, Peters H, Granger M, Chunekamrai N: Clin Chem 14:1033–1065, 1968)

TABLE 15-8. PREPARATION OF REAGENTS

Reagent	Preparation and use
Ninhydrin (Nin)	2 g ninhydrin (1,2,3-triketohydrindene hydrate) 50 ml ethanol (95%) 100 ml water 850 ml n-butanol Stable for 2–4 wk at room temp. Spray chromatogram and heat at 85–90° for 8–10 min.
Isatin	1 g isatin 20 ml acetic acid 480 ml ethanol (95%) Store in refrigerator. Stable for 2–4 wk. Spray chromatogram and heat at 90° for 10 min.
Toluidine blue (CSA)	1.2 g toluidine blue 800 ml acetone 200 ml water Stable at room temp.
Sulfanilic acid	4.5 g sulfanilic acid 45 ml conc hydrochloric acid 100 ml water Warm to dissolve and then add 355 ml water. Use as described below. Stable at room temp.
Diazotized sulfanilic acid (DSA)	2.2 g sodium nitrate 50 ml water Chill sodium nitrite for 10 min in ice bath or freezer. Chill 50 ml sulfanilic acid. Combine cold solutions and chill for additional 15 min. The diazotized reagent is stable for 2–4 days in refrigerator. For spray reagent, combine equal parts of DSA and cold 10% (w/v) potassium carbonate; use immediately.
p-Anisidine (p-Anis)	0.2% (w/v) p-anisidine in ethanol (95%) Stable for 2–4 wk in refrigerator. Spray chromatogram and heat at 110–120° for 8 min.
Bromcresol green (BCG)	0.2 g bromcresol green (sodium salt may be used) 500 ml ethanol (95%) Neutralize with 1 N sodium hydroxide until color changes to green blue when tested on filter paper. Stable at room temp.
Ferricyanide–nitroprusside	1 g sodium hydroxide dissolved in 10 ml water 1 g sodium nitroprusside dissolved in 10 ml water 1 g potassium ferricyanide dissolved in 10 ml water Salts are dissolved separately and then combined. Mixture is diluted with 90 ml water. After standing for about 20 min, initial dark color changes to pale yellow and is ready to use. Stable for 2–4 wk in refrigerator.

TABLE 15-8. PREPARATION OF REAGENTS *(continued)*

Reagent	Preparation and use
Dichloroquinonechlorimide (DCC)	1 gm. dichloroquinonechlorimide in 100 ml ethanol (95%) Spray lightly but evenly on both sides and allow to dry. Overspray with solution of 0.5% (w/v) sodium tetraborate in water. DCC solution is stable for 1–2 wk in refrigerator. Borate solution is stable 2–4 mo in refrigerator.
Aniline phthalate	8.5 g phthalic anhydride 25 ml ethanol (95%) 50 ml water 425 ml n-butanol 5 ml aniline Let stand overnight in refrigerator before use. Stable for 2–4 wk in refrigerator. Spray chromatogram and heat at 110° for 10 min.
Naphthoresorcinol	0.2% (w/v) naphthoresorcinol in ethanol (95%) 8.5% (v/v) ortho phosphoric acid Immediately before use combine 1 volume phosphoric acid with 5 volumes naphthoresorcinol. Spray chromatogram and heat for 10 min at 90° in oven containing pan of water.
p-Dimethylaminobenzaldehyde (PDAB)	2 g p-dimethylaminobenzaldehyde 10 ml conc hydrochloric acid Dissolve before adding 90 m water. Stable 1–2 wk in refrigerator.
p- Dimethylaminocinnamaldehyde	0.5 g p-dimethylaminocinnamaldehyde Dissolve in 20 ml conc hydrochloric acid. Dilute to 200 ml with water. Stable 4–6 mo in refrigerator.
Iodine–azide	50 ml 0.1 N iodine (aqueous solution prepared using potassium iodide) 50 ml ethanol (95%) 1.5 g sodium azide is dissolved in above mixture. Stable approx 1 wk in refrigerator.

(Berry HK, Leonard C, Peters H, Granger M, Chunekamrai N: Clin Chem 14:1033–1065, 1968)

TABLE 15-9. REACTIONS OF VARIOUS SUGARS WITH THREE COMMON REAGENTS

	Combistix	Galatest	Anthrone
Glucose	+	+	+
Galactose	−	+	+
Fructose	−	+	+
Lactose	−	+	+
Sucrose	−	−	+

(Berry HK, Leonard C, Peters H, Granger M, Chunekamrai N: Clin Chem 14:1033–1065, 1968

The 2,4-dinitrophenylhydrazine test is positive with keto acids such as phenylpyruvic acid; pyruvic acid; α-ketoglutaric acid; keto acids derived from leucine, valine, and isoleucine; diacetic acid; and large quantities of acetone. With chromatography, the keto acid in a specimen having a positive reaction can be identified; α-ketoglutaric acid is most often responsible for a positive reaction (8).

Millon's reagent shows a strongly positive reaction with tyrosine, *p*-hydroxyphenylacetic, *p*-hydroxyphenylpyruvic, and *p*-hydroxyphenyllactic acid. Millon's reagent test is useful in rapid testing of specimens from infants with suspected tyrosinosis or in checking for ascorbic acid deficiency in infants (8).

Whereas paper chromatography was originally used to identify amino acids in urine, current methodology is primarily separation by thin-layer chromatography. Berry's method (7) is as follows:

Thin-layer chromatography of eluates of dried blood specimens has the capability of revealing relatively small increases above normal of leucine, phenylalanine, methionine, tyrosine, proline, and histidine. Amino acids are eluted from uniform discs of dried blood with 70% ethanol by overnight extraction in the cold. The eluates are streaked on commercially prepared plates of microcrystalline cellulose. The plates are developed twice in a solvent system containing *n*-butanol, acetone, acetic acid, water (35:35:10:20). During the second run, Ninhydrin reagent is added directly to the solvent mixture, thereby ensuring uniform development.

SCREENING FOR DISORDERS

Alkaptonuria

Alkaptonuria is a defect in the body's ability to metabolize tyrosine and phenylalanine, resulting in the formation of the intermediary product homogentisic acid (2:5 dihydroxylphenylacetic acid). This substance is excreted in the urine and turns black when oxidized through exposure to the oxygen of the air. Homogentisic acid may be deposited in cartilaginous tissues, where it is slowly oxidized to a dark color, producing the pathologic condition known as ochronosis.

Methods of detection are as follows:

1. Ferric chloride test. Upon the addition of dilute ferric chloride solution, a deep blue color appears for a moment until oxidation is complete.
2. Alkali test. The addition of NaOH 10% to alkaptonuric urine produces a brown color in 1–2 min.
3. Benedict's qualitative test. The technique is the same as that for sugar in the urine. The reduction is atypical, ending in a brown to black color. (Clinitest is not interfered with by homogentisic acid and therefore cannot be used for this test.)
4. Film test. Alkaptonuric urine blackens sensitized photographic film (hydroquinine reaction). Place an aliquot of alkaline urine with 0.1 N NaOH added on photographic sensitive paper. The photographic presumptive test includes alkalating the urine, which rapidly oxidizes to dark brown to black on standing.
5. Enzyme. The enzyme homogentisic acid oxidase is used for quantification by the method of Metz, described by Sommerfelt (56) and the method of Seegmiller (50).

Cystinuria

Another error of protein metabolism involves cystine. The condition results in the appearance of large quantities of the colorless, hexagonal crystals of cystine in the urine *i.e.*,—cystinuria.

One congenital defect in renal reabsorption of cystine, lysine, arginine, and ornithine predisposes an individual to renal calculi. In cystinosis, also congenital, cystine crystals are deposited in many tissues and organs, and there is usually associated an increased excretion of all amino acids in the urine along with impairment of other renal functions. These patients usually die at an early age due to renal failure.

Besides identification of cystine crystals, cystine can be detected chemically by reduction with cyanide to cysteine, which then reacts with nitroprusside to produce a red color. Reagents for this are as follows:

1. Sodium cyanide 5%. Dissolve 1 g NaCn in water (*Caution*: This is poisonous.) Prepare fresh.
2. Sodium nitroprusside 5%. Dissolve 1 g sodium nitroprusside (nitroferricyanide) in 20 ml water. Prepare fresh.

The procedure is as follows:

1. To 5 ml urine add 2 ml NaCN 5%. (Do not pipette by mouth.) Mix.

2. Let stand for 10 min.
3. Add five drops of fresh sodium nitroprusside 5%. Mix. Normal urines show a pale brown or occasionally faint flesh color; with cystinuric urines, a magenta color is obtained. (This color may fade.)

The urine must be free of protein. If necessary, add a little acetic acid, heat to boiling, and filter.

Glycinuria

Glycinuria is associated with calcium oxalate renal stones and excessive secretion of glycine. Sulfite oxidase deficiency shows a large peak of cysteic acid, which can be identified as sulfocysteine due to the sulfite oxidase catalyzing reaction. Other related diseases include β-mercaptolactate-cysteine disulfiduria. Also isovalericacidemia and β-hydroxyisovalericaciduria are related. Methylmalonicacid may be excreted.

The thiosulfate test for glycinuria is performed by adding a drop of sodium azide 3% in 0.1 N iodine (W/V) to a drop of urine in a porcelain dish. A positive test, such as bubbling and discoloration, is the indication of sulfite oxidase deficiency. The patient with sulfite oxidase deficiency excretes large amounts of thiosulfate, sulfite, and s-sulfocysteine. Since sulfite is unstable, the presence of thiosulfate may prove to be more reliable in making the diagnosis (25).

Histidinemia

The excretion of histidine is due to the enzyme defect of hepatic histidase. The clinical picture includes speech defect and mental retardation. The ferric chloride test for PKU may well be positive with histidinemia due to imidazole pyruvic acid in the urine. Chromatographic analysis of blood is necessary to distinguish between various aminoacidemias.

Hyperoxaluria

Hyperoxaluria is a disorder of oxalate metabolism with recurrent calcium oxalate stones in the kidney and with oxalate crystals in the urine. Oxalate crystals may be frequently seen in the urine of normal persons, but not in excessive quantities.

Hypervalinemia

Valine appears increased specifically due to an absence of valine transaminase and results in mental retardation (23).

Hyperprolinemia

In hyperprolinemia proline oxidase is abnormal, and the amino acid proline appears in increased quantities. Patients exhibit a photogenic epilepsy, deafness, and mental retardation. An associated disease is *hydroxyprolinemia*, which is a hydroxyproline oxidase defect resulting in similar retardation and microscopic hematuria (23).

The Joseph's Syndrome

The Joseph's syndrome is associated with increased proline, hydroxyproline, and excretion of glycine in the urine and is often also associated with convulsions (23).

Homocystinuria

Cystathionine synthase deficiency results in increased methionine and homocysteine (Fig. 15–1). Mental retardation, along with thromboembolic phenomena, dislocated lenses, and homocystine in the urine are typical (23).

There is a silver–nitroprusside test for homocysteine. To 5 ml salt-saturated urine in a test tube add 0.5 ml silver nitrate 1% in ammonia 3%. To a control test tube add urine sample and 0.5 ml ammonia 3% without silver nitrate. After 1 min, add 0.5 ml nitroprusside solution 1% to each of the test tubes. An immediate purple color indicates the presence of homocysteine. Cystines do not react in this test (57).

Cystathioninuria

This has been associated with mental retardation and has a deficiency of cystathionidase.

β-aminoisobutyricaciduria

Other defined entities include β-aminoisobutyricaciduria, in which patients excrete β-aminoisobutyric acid but have no apparent physical abnormalities (26).

Maple Syrup Urine Disease

Maple syrup urine disease involves abnormalities of valine, leucine, and isoleucine metabolism. The basic block is the failure of oxidative decarboxylation of keto acids, which causes increased levels of amino acids

Fig. 15-1. Abbreviated scheme of sulfur metabolism. Dietary sulfur enters as methionine and cysteine (or the oxidized form, cystine). (Frimpter GW: N Engl J Med 289 (16): 835–841, 1973)

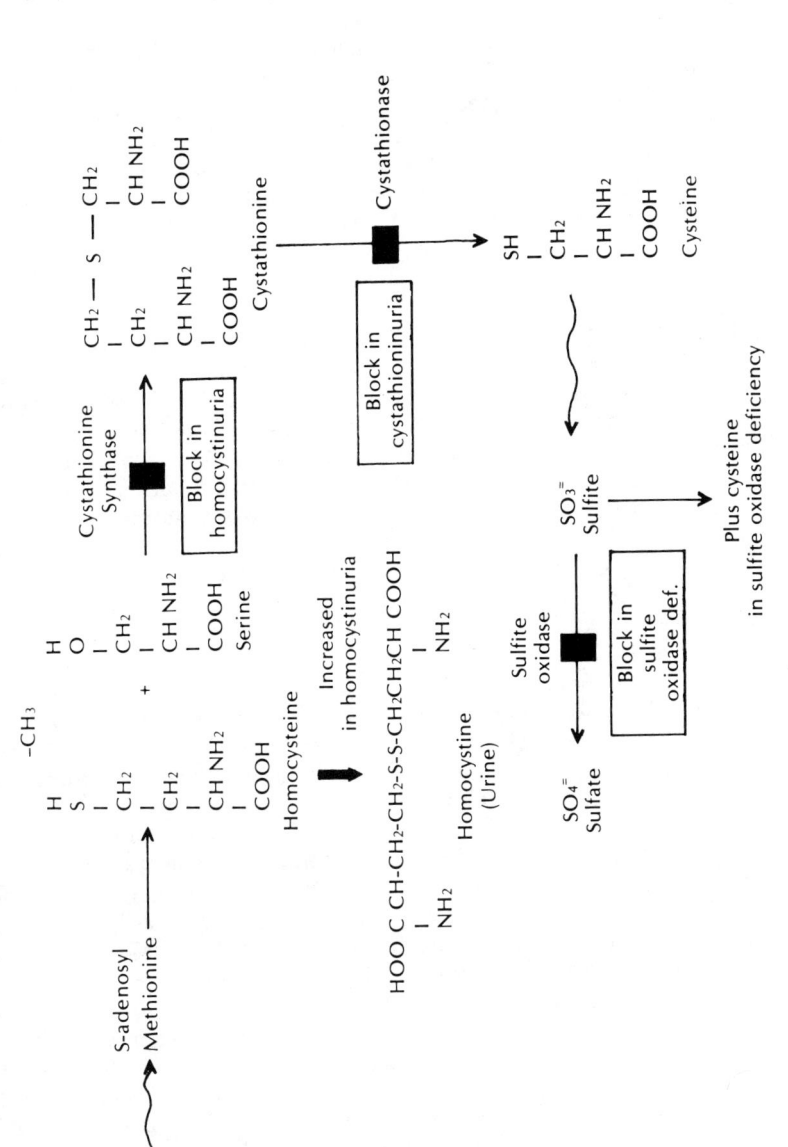

and their keto derivatives in plasma and in urine. In such cases large amounts of both keto acids and nonketo acids with the properties of α-hydroxy acids are excreted in the urine. The hydroxy acids impart an odor of maple syrup, from whence came the name of the disease. Gross mental retardation results, and death occurs before the age of 2 years. Finding large amounts of valine, leucine, and isoleucine on two-dimensional chromatography of the urine in a mentally retarded child is diagnostic.

Phenylketonuria

Normally 80% of dietary phenylalanine is converted to tyrosine. However, in phenylketonuria the deficiency of the liver enzyme phenylalanine hydroxylase prevents the normal transformation of phenylalanine to tyrosine. Phenylalanine becomes elevated in the blood and appears in the urine together with other abnormal metabolic products (26). These include phenylpyruvic acid, phenylacetic acid, phenylacetylglutamine, and ortho-hydroxyphenylacetic acid. During pregnancy, the mother performs the hydroxylation of phenylalanine for the fetus; it is only after birth that blood levels of phenylalanine increase in newborns with this metabolic defect. Phenylalanine at a blood level of 10 mg/dl or greater exerts a deleterious effect on the brain that results in mental retardation. At a level of 10 mg/dl blood metabolites of phenylalanine, *i.e.*, phenylpyruvic acid and phenylacetic acid, appear in the urine (47). Untreated phenylketonuric children develop intelligence quotients that range from 10 to about 50 (46). This severe mental deterioration is preventable if the condition is recognized and dietary restriction of phenylalanine is carried out until the child develops alternative metabolic pathways to handle this amino acid.

Since as many as 1% of mentally defective persons may be phenylketonuric (46) and adequate dietary care can prevent mental deterioration, there is a great urgency for early detection of this metabolic defect. In fact, many states have laws that require the testing of all newborns for the defect. Various tests are available for detecting this condition, including direct quantification of the level of phenylalanine in the blood; a semi-quantitative measurement can be made by the bacterial inhibition Guthrie test. A simple qualitative test may be made using reagent strips impregnated with ferric chloride and glacial acetic acid. As recommended by Baird (3), the reagent strip can be moistened with urine via contact with a wet diaper and the results read according to the color changes effected. A green, gray, or dark blue color developing within 60 sec is considered positive. Such reagent strips are commercially available from several manufacturers, *e.g.*, Phenistix from Ames Laboratories.

In order for any law or medical regimen to be effective in preventing mental retardation from this metabolic defect, one point must be kept in mind. All tests for the presence of this condition may be negative for several days and for as long as 3 weeks after birth. Testing for this defect should be as much a pediatric as an obstetric responsibility. By using reagent strips, the mother can easily make the test after returning home from the hospital. Measurement of the orthohydroxyphenylacetic acid can be determined easily in urine by both biochemical and microbiologic tests. The incidence is about 1:40,000 births, and the common test is the PKU procedure.

The urine from a phenylketonuria patient gives a green color with a ferric chloride solution. The Guthrie test is most commonly used and is performed 3–5 days after birth. It is a microbiologic assay which measures the ability of the patient's blood to inhibit the growth of *Bacillus subtilis* by β-thienylalanine, which is an antagonist to phenylalanine. The test is performed as follows:

1. Small paper disks impregnated with the patient's blood from a heel puncture are placed on the screening plate on which the bacteria are growing.
2. Phenylalanine from blood diffuses into the media and reverses the inhibition of β-thienylalanine.
3. Semiquantification occurs through use of disks containing known phenylalanine amounts.
4. Quantities are interpolated. False-negative tests occur in patients being treated with antibiotics to which *B. subtilis* is sensitive.

Tyrosinosis

Tyrosinosis is due to a defect of enzymes with excretion of large quantities of *p*-hydroxyphenylpyruvic acid. The deficiency is due to the *p*-hydroxyphenylpyruvic acid oxidase enzyme and can be detected by the use of Millon's reagent (Table 15-7) or paper chromatography.

Neonatal tyrosinemia is the most frequent finding in mass surveys of newborn infants. Approximately 0.5%–1% of all newborns and 25% of premature infants have elevated concentrations of tyrosine during the first week of life. The elevations of tyrosine are accompanied by elevation of phenylalanine, leading to positive tests for phenylalanine in routine screening (7).

The nitrosonapthol test for tyrosinemia is performed as follows. To 1 ml 2.63 N nitric acid, add one drop of sodium nitrite solution (2.5% in water) and then 10 drops of nitrosonapthol reagent (0.1% in 95% ethylalcohol). Add three drops of urine and mix. The formation of an orange red color indicates the presence of excessive metabolites of tyrosine such as *p*-hydroxyphenol, *p*-hydroxypyruvic acid, and *p*-hydroxyphenylacetic acid (44).

Other Metabolic Errors

The urea cycle metabolic errors involving ornithine, citrulline, argininosuccinic acid, and arginase with various enzyme blocks can result in a carbamylphosphate synthetase deficiency and an ornithine transcarbamylase deficiency, producing citrullinemia and argininosuccinicaciduria.

Hyperlysinemia and saccharopinuria are common. Saccharopine has been shown to be an intermediary product of lysine metabolism and to be associated with mentally retarded patients who have a deficiency of an enzyme, aminoadipic semialdehyde–glutamate reductase.

Other aminoacidurias include hyper-β-alaninemia, carnosinemia, and hypersarcosinemia (26).

16 Screening for Diseases, Drugs, or Poisons

If a screening test is to be used on a large scale, it must be not only effective but economical. If a test is initiated by a physician, it is important that the clinical information relating to possible inborn errors of metabolism be known for proper interpretation; the abnormality should be sought through a review of the natural history of the disease, its prevalence, genetic influence, and methods for detection. The largest group of metabolic errors includes those which are of genetic origin (see Ch. 15, Generalized Metabolic Derangements.) However, a routine screening by urinalysis should be done in all infants.

PEDIATRIC SCREENING FOR DISEASE

The method described by Bradley (11) several years ago still has usefulness and is reproduced for its clarity.

1. *Screening for bacteriuria.* If only one specimen is available for complete urinalysis this should be done first. Alternative procedures include a Gram stain of the uncentrifuged, well mixed specimen and the quantitative loop culture method or a miniculture method, all of which require a drop or two of urine. The tetrazolium reduction test, a simpler test, is used for mass screening and requires 2 ml urine.

2. *Specific gravity.* At this point a drop may be used for refractometer estimation of specific gravity.
3. *Chemical screening (basic).* Using combination reagent strips, dip and read for all or some of the following.

```
pH      ⎫
protein ⎪
glucose ⎬  e.g., Labstix*    ⎫
ketone  ⎪                    ⎪
blood   ⎭                    ⎬  e.g., Bili-labstix*
bilirubin                    ⎪
urobilinogen, e.g., Urobilistix*  ⎭
```

If the combined Bili-labstix is not to be used, Ictotest* for bilirubin is as simple and is easier to interpret than Bilistix reagent strips. The use of reagent strips makes it more certain that tests will be done because of the ease of operation.

4. *Test for copper-reducing substances.* It is most important that this test be performed on all infant specimens by either the Benedict or Clinitest* tablet method. The test should be done when the glucose oxidase test is positive to distinguish higher levels of glucose (Table 16-1). The test requires 5 drops of urine.

At this point the specimen should be centrifuged in a disposable centrifuge tube, and the clear supernatant separated from the sediment and refrigerated.

5. *The sediment.* A drop of the concentrated sediment is examined under a coverslip for red blood cells, leukocytes, renal epithelial cells, casts, and excessive numbers of crystals. These are usually graded as to number of cells in an average of 10 high power fields.

Alternatively the uncentrifuged, well mixed specimen may be examined in a counting chamber and reported as cells per cubic millimeter. The distinguishing of renal epithelial cells from polymorphonuclear leukocytes is aided by staining.

*Ames Company, Elkhart, Indiana.

TABLE 16-1. SENSITIVITY OF TESTS FOR GLUCOSE AND REDUCING SUBSTANCES IN URINE

Benedict's Cu reduction	Usual qualitative interpretation	Neg.	Trace	1+	2+	3+	4+
	Approx mg/dl	0	10–100	250	500–1000	2000	4000
Clinitest* Cu reduction	Usual qualitative interpretation	—	—	Trace	1+ 2+	3+	4+
	Approx mg/dl	0	—	250	500 750	1000	2000
Glucose oxidase reagent strip†	Usual qualitative interpretation	"Light"..........."Dark"...........					
	Approx mg/dl	0	40–100	250	500+		

*Ames Co., Elkhart, Indiana.
†Sensitivity in glucose in water as low as 3 mg/dl; therefore is more sensitive in dilute urines.
(Bradley MD: Hum Pathol 2(2):309–320, 1971)

6. *The supernatant.* The supernatant is used for the following tests:
    a. A confirmatory protein test using 1 ml urine and 3 drops of sulfosalicylic acid 20% is performed and the results graded by turbidity.
    b. Separation of sugars is carried out by thin-layer chromatography when Benedict's test is positive and the glucose oxidase test negative.
7. *Amino acids.* Screening for amino acids requires a greater volume of urine. This may be collected separately from that used in the basic screening procedure. Both the laboratory and clinical interpretations of these tests require care, and the pathologist may prefer screening by a one-way paper chromatographic test, or he may set up two-dimensional paper chromatography.
    a. The *ferric chloride test* requires 1–2 ml urine. Ferric chloride 10% is added drop by drop; a color appears within 30 sec (Table 15-6). There are many color changes with substances other than amino acids that may invalidate results.
    b. *2,4-Dinitrophenylhydrazine* (DPNH), 0.1% in 2 N hydrochloric acid, is added to an equal volume of urine. A white yellow precipitate forms in 2–3 min. The yellow hydrazones of keto acids may be further extracted (Table 15-6).
    c. The *cyanide–nitroprusside test* for cystinuria. Five milliliters of urine is required for this test, although a spot test may be used. A 2-ml portion of freshly prepared sodium cyanide 5% is added to urine made alkaline and allowed to stand for 10 min. Five drops of sodium nitroprusside 5% is added and the solution mixed. A purplish magenta color is seen with cystine (Table 15-6). Hexagonal cystine crystals may be seen in the sediment examination.
8. *Test for excessive mucopolysaccharides.* This test requires 5 ml fresh urine at room temperature (cold urine will give a positive test). One milliliter of cetyltrimethylammonium bromide (CTAB) 5% in 1M citrate buffer at pH 6 is added to the urine and mixed well. A heavy flocculent precipitate at 30 min is positive for gargoylism and for some disorders of connective tissue, such as the Marfan and Morquio–Ullrich syndromes. An alternative is the paper spot test (Table 16-2).

    Tests for melituria, amino acids, and mucopolysaccharides may be grouped as a selective screening procedure for infants with failure to thrive, mental deficiency, or neurologic deficit. Additional tests that could be added to the battery include the metachromatic stain of the urinary sediment for metachromatic leukodystrophy, which requires 15 ml urine.
9. *Screening for lead poisoning.* In screening for lead poisoning, a test for urinary delta aminolevulinic acid (ALA) may be performed, using a disposable plastic chromatography column containing ion exchange resin. This test requires 0.5 ml urine. An alternative procedure uses high voltage electrophoresis and thin-layer chromatography. Great accuracy in the demonstration of urinary lead is possible with the technique, which employs bismuth as a lead coprecipitant and atomic absorption spectroscopy. The complexity of present methods for lead determination, however, makes it apparent that they cannot be regarded readily as screening tests in the sense that the term has been used in this review.

In addition to specific diseases resulting from inborn metabolism errors, genetic diseases of the kidney may be identified early in life through urinary findings (Table 16-3). Hematuria is seen with Alport's syndrome of hereditary nephritis as well as in acute childhood nephritis or in coagulation defects. Functional genetic abnormalities may be associated with a

TABLE 16-2. URINARY SCREENING TESTS FOR INBORN ERRORS OF METABOLISM

	Copper reduction test	CTAB* test	Metachromatic stain
Phenylketonuria	±	–	–
Tyrosinuria	±	–	–
Galactosemia	+	–	–
Fructosuria	+	–	–
Alkaptonuria	+	–	–
Hurler's syndrome	–	+	–
Morquio-Ullrich syndrome	–	+	–
Marfan's syndrome	–	±	–
Metachromatic leukodystrophy	–	–	+
Tay-Sachs disease	–	–	±

*Cetyltrimethylammonium bromide.
(Bradley MD: Hum Pathol 2(2):309–320, 1971)

TABLE 16-3. SOME GENETIC KIDNEY DISEASES WITH URINARY FINDINGS

Structural defects*	Functional defects†
Nephritis—various, e.g., Alport's syndrome	Cystinuria
	Dibasic aminoaciduria
Familial Mediterranean fever with amyloidosis	Renal glycosuria
Fabry's disease	Glucose-galactose malabsorption
Infantile polycystic disease	Hartnup disease
Medullary cystic disease	Iminoglycinuria
Infantile nephrosis	Fanconi syndrome
Unilateral hydronephrosis	Proximal renal tubular acidosis
Megaureter and other urinary tract anomalies	Distal renal tubular acidosis
Nail patella syndrome	Vasopressin-resistant diabetes insipidus

*Findings include proteinuria, hematuria, increased leukocytes or renal epithelial cells, and associated bacteriuria.
†Findings include the amino acids and sugars mentioned, polyuria, elevated pH. Some nonrenal diseases such as galactosemia induce proteinuria and aminoaciduria. Oxalosis may lead to obstruction and renal failure.
(Bradley MD: Hum Pathol 2(2):309–320, 1971)

transport defect of the proximal renal tubular epithelial cell. The aminoacidurias include glucosurias and cystinurias as well as familial renal glucosuria. Hartnup disease with glucoglycinuria and the rare proximal renal tubular acidosis seen in male infants may be recognized. Urinary pH may be very high, as seen with the distal renal tubular acidosis. Recently a screening test for urinary δ-aminolevulinic acid has been devised that uses resin-impregnated paper for the collection of urine (60).

SCREENING FOR DRUG ABUSE

Drug abuse testing in human urine is a major and fast-growing laboratory activity. In the determination of any drug for a toxicologic reason, there must be a quality control of the specificity: the testing procedure must be specific to identify the drug, and its concentration limits must be known. In addition, the method used to detect such a drug must have a sensitivity to the drug which indicates a minimal, acceptable, lower level of concentration in the urine. False-positive and false-negative detections have great legal significance, and persons may be imprisoned for an erroneous test result. Methods employed include thin-layer chromatography, gas–liquid chromatography, radioimmunoassay, enzyme immunoassay, and others. This testing is a special branch of toxicology, which may become a subsection of activities in the urinalysis laboratory (18).

17 Functional Tests

PHYSIOLOGIC BASIS FOR FUNCTIONAL TESTS

All the cells of the body are wholly dependent upon the kidney to create for them an environment that is relatively constant in its ionic composition and its extracellular volume. This complete dependence of all other organs for ionic homeostasis places a burden upon the proper functioning of the kidneys not only for well-being but for actual existence. There is, quite rationally, a deep concern whenever the functional capacity of the kidneys is jeopardized.

The adequacy of renal function is determined by the measurement of the composition of the extracellular fluid (plasma) and the clinical assessment of the volume of the extracellular fluid. These clinical and laboratory tests are much more effective in evaluating the extent of impairment of kidney function than is the examination of the urine. However, examination of the urine may be of critical importance as the first indicator of kidney disease.

In order to accept the fact that routine urinalysis does not measure renal function and to appreciate the rationale for renal function tests, the mechanisms of kidney function must be understood. How does the kidney create and maintain a constant internal environment in the presence of mechanisms that continuously pour in a vast number of differing types and quantities of substances? What are the mechanisms whereby nonessential and noxious metabolites are removed and the essential metabolites retained in spite of the fact they are intermingled in the same medium? If the various mechanisms employed by the kidney are known, then various challenging tests can be devised to measure each individual and separate capacity.

Strong evidence exists to support concepts developed by various physiologists, such as Richards (48) and Smith (54,55), that extracellular fluid homeostasis is in part maintained in man by the kidney. The kidney contributes to the maintenance of homeostasis through three processes: 1) glomerular filtration, 2) tubular secretion, and 3) tubular reabsorption. Blood reaches the glomeruli of the kidney by passing through the glomerular capillary. Under normal circumstances, the red blood cells, protein, and larger molecules in the blood remain on the blood side of the glomerular membrane while the pressure within the glomerular blood vessel forces water and small molecules (such as sodium, chloride, creatinine, urea, etc.) across the membrane. The normal kidney contains 1 million such glomeruli; hence, there are 2 million glomeruli in the normal human.

The amount of glomerular filtrate (the fluid formed by the passage of water and chemicals across the glomerular membrane) is surprisingly large—150 liters/day. The normal individual only excretes 1 liter urine per day so that 149 liters must be reabsorbed; in addition, the chemical substances passing through the glomerular membrane that are necessary for the maintenance of homeostasis must be reabsorbed, while those which are undesirable must be excreted. Some chemical substances which are not processed by glomerular filtration also need to be excreted from the body. These are secreted into the tubule. The 150 liters of glomerular filtrate that are formed each day are processed by tubular reabsorption and tubular secretion.

The composition of the fluid crossing the glomerular membrane is identical to that of plasma for low-molecular-weight substances; for example, the concentration of sodium in the plasma is the same as it is in the glomerular filtrate. One can easily see that, if 150 liters of glomerular filtrate are formed each day and the sodium concentration of the patient's plasma is 135 mEq/liter, the total amount of sodium filtered is 20,250 mEq/24 hour (the product of 150×135). If this sodium chloride were passed into the final urine, the individual would quickly die of salt depletion. By a process of tubular reabsorption, approximately 99.5% of the filtered sodium is reabsorbed.

Not all the chemicals present in the glomerular filtrate are desirable for the body. Such substances as urea, creatinine, uric acid, and other substances must be excreted by the kidney. Most of these substances are filtered at the glomerulus; in addition, some are secreted by the tubules into the glomerular filtrate. Little, if any, reabsorption of most of these chemicals occurs; most, if not all, of what has been filtered plus what is secreted will ultimately appear in the urine. Hence, the kidney maintains the homeostasis of the ionic composition of the body fluids by reabsorbing the needed chemicals and substances and ultimately excreting the unwanted and undesirable substances.

The kidney also performs the complex job of maintaining the total volume of fluid within the body. By the reception of a variety of signals from the brain, heart, and glands (such as the adrenal gland, which is the site of aldosterone production, and the hypothalamus-posterior pituitary, which is the site of antidiuretic hormone production) the kidney senses the need for excreting smaller or larger amounts of fluid thus varying the urine output from as low as 0.5 liters/day to greater than 2–3 liters/day.

Tests of renal function are designed to evaluate the process of glomerular filtration and the ultimate retention of substances desired for the body's economy and the excretion of unwanted substances. These tests specifically examine the adequacy of glomerular filtration and the extent of tubular reabsorption and tubular secretion. Renal function can be measured at several levels. Reasonably adequate estimations of renal function can be determined by the examination of certain plasma chemistries (blood urea nitrogen and creatinine), but the precise measurement of renal function requires the quantification of certain excreted substances which are known to be handled exclusively by mechanisms of glomerular filtration, tubular secretion, or tubular reabsorption. These techniques often require the collection of urine samples over a timed interval, the accurate measurement of the volume of urine, and the concurrent sampling of the patient's plasma. As a consequence, except in specialized situations, these measurements are not routinely available from the laboratory.

MEASUREMENT OF GLOMERULAR FILTRATION RATE

The glomerular filtration rate indicates the capability of the kidney to rid the body of unwanted substances. Many substances pass through the glomerular membrane with reasonable ease, especially if the molecules are relatively small, and then find themselves in the tubular lumen. In general, unwanted substances are not subjected to any reabsorptive process but remain in the tubular urine as it is progressively processed by the kidney. While these unwanted substances remain, the substances necessary for homeostasis are reabsorbed.

The quantitative measurement of the capacity for glomerular filtration is referred to as a clearance. Clearance might best be understood as the amount of the substance which is removed from a volume of blood as it passes through the glomerulus (Fig. 17–1). The substances removed have crossed the glomerular capillary membrane and now appear in the tubular fluid (ultimately the urine). The amount of these substances appearing in the urine over a period of time, divided by the plasma concentration of the substance as it goes into the kidney, represents the calculation of clearance. The clearance therefore represents the quantitative removal of a certain amount of an identifiable substance from a specific volume of blood over an interval of time so that, when it is reported in units as ml/min or liter/24 hours, the clearance term represents the volume of blood totally cleared of this particular substance over the time interval indicated.

Those who develop an appreciation of the concept of clearance will better understand renal function and functional test methods. Part of the difficulty in understanding lies in the fact that, although clearance relates to the ability of the kidney to excrete a substance, it nevertheless is measured and reported in terms of milliliters of plasma per minute. Clearance is defined as that volume of plasma which contains the precise amount of the substance being studied that is excreted in the urine in 1 min

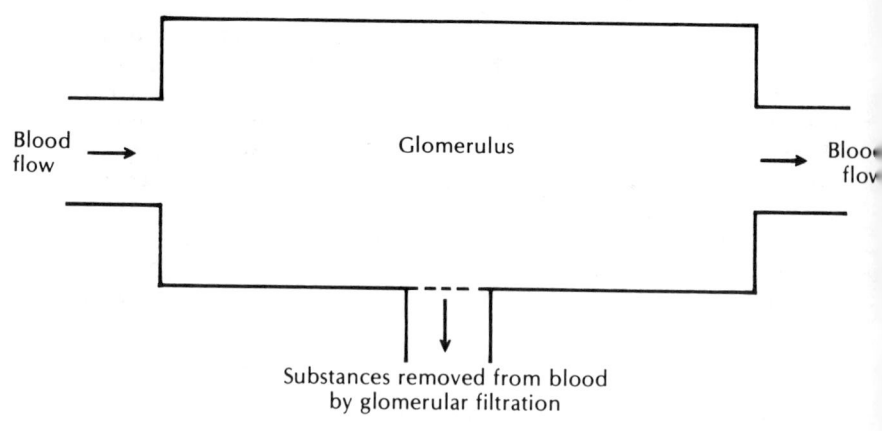

Fig. 17–1. As blood flows through the glomerulus, it loses a certain amount of the substances which it contained prior to entering (such as urea and creatinine).

of time. (The unit of time has been arbitrarily selected; the usual time is per minute or per day.) This may be readily appreciated by the following example.

If a patient has a urea concentration of 10 mg/dl plasma and excretes 10 mg urea in urine in 1 min, 100 ml plasma has been cleared of all its contained urea in 1 min of time, *i.e.*, clearance for urea would be 100 ml plasma per minute. This may be expressed as

$$C_x = \frac{U_x V}{P_x}$$

where

C = clearance
x = substance for which the clearance is being determined (urea, creatinine)
U_x = urine concentration of substance x per milliliter
V = volume of urine excreted per minute in milliliters
P_x = plasma concentration of substance x per milliliter

The ideal substance to measure glomerular filtration rate is one that is completely filtered at the glomerular capillary membrane and then is not subjected to either tubular secretion or reabsorption. No substance naturally occurring in the body fulfills these restrictions, but creatinine comes close. Creatinine is primarily filtered at the glomerulus; an additional quantity of creatinine (rarely exceeding 20% of the total) is added by tubular excretion. Creatinine clearance represents the easiest mechanism for the measurement of glomerular filtration because it is produced within the body and most is excreted by glomerular filtration. More accurate measurements of glomerular filtration rate can be performed by using such substances as inulin or iothalamate. Both of these substances are freely filtered at the glomerulus but are not subjected to either tubular secretion or reabsorption so that the total amount filtered at the glomerulus ultimately appears in the urine. These substances can be administered to the individual and serve as ideal markers of glomerular filtration rate.

TWENTY-FOUR HOUR CREATININE CLEARANCE

A 24-hour period of collection presumes that the patient's glomerular filtration rate is relatively constant throughout the 24 hours of collection. The determination is made as follows:

1. Collect urine for a 24-hour period. The patient voids at 8:00 A.M. but discards the urine; from that point on, all the urine is saved until 8:00 A.M. the following morning, at which time the patient completes the collection by voiding and adding this last urine to the 24-hour collection.
2. Collect a plasma sample at 8:00 P.M. (midway through the collection period), or practical conditions may dictate that the specimen be collected at the end of the collection period.
3. Measure the total volume of urine and urine creatinine.
4. Analyze the plasma for creatinine.
5. Calculate the creatinine clearance.

SHORT-TERM CREATININE CLEARANCE

The short-term creatinine clearance test is performed over a shorter interval of time, usually varying from 30 min to 4 hours. Ideally, the urine flow rate should be about 5 ml/min (300 cc/hour); this can be accomplished by the oral administration of 1000–2000 ml water preceding the test. This test presumes constancy of glomerular filtration rate over the time of collection. The short-term creatinine clearance is determined as follows:

1. Collect a urine sample over an arbitrarily chosen period of time. The patient, if medically appropriate, should imbibe 1000–2000 ml water before the test is begun. Accurate timing is critically important. For example, have the patient drink 1500 ml water from 9:15 A.M. until 10:00 A.M. At 10:00 A.M., have the patient void and discard the urine. Collect all the urine formed from 10:00 A.M. until 12:00 noon. Have the patient void at 12:00 noon and save.
2. Collect a plasma sample midway through the collection period, *i.e.*, at

11:00 A.M. Follow steps 3 through 5 as described for the 24-hour creatinine clearance determination.

IOTHALAMATE CLEARANCE

Iothalamate is handled exclusively by glomerular filtration. The isotope (^{125}I iothalamate) may be administered by continuous infusion, by subcutaneous injection, or by a single intravenous injection. The detailed method for the subcutaneous injection technique follows.

Glomerular filtration rate may be measured by injecting the patient with Glofil-^{125}I (sodium iothalamate ^{125}I)* and collecting both blood and urine samples at regular intervals. The renal clearance of Glofil-^{125}I closely approximates that of inulin, but the radioactive Glofil-^{125}I has the advantage of being easily measured whereas inulin requires a tedious colorimetric determination.

Reagents and equipment required are as follows.

1. Glofil-^{125}I, about 20 microcuries added to 0.1 ml 1:1000 aqueous epinephrine.
2. Sterile, disposable (tuberculin) syringe for injecting Glofil-^{125}I and epinephrine.
3. Suitable urine collection containers and heparinized blood-collecting tubes.
4. Disposable volumetric pipettes, 1 ml.
5. Scintillation well counter.

Procedure

To reduce unnecessary radiation of the thyroid, it is recommended that the patient be given orally 10 drops of Lugol's solution in a glass of water the evening prior to the study. No diet or water restriction is necessary. Oral water load of 20 ml/kg body weight is given to initiate a diuresis, and throughout the study urinary output is replaced with water.

Testing procedure is as follows:

1. Prior to injection of Glofil, have the patient empty the bladder. Save this sample and label it "background sample."
2. Carefully inject 20 microcuries of Glofil-^{125}I mixed with epinephrine subcutaneously in the deltoid area.
3. Equilibrate 40–60 min and then have the patient void and discard.
4. Note the exact time and begin the first time-clearance period of 30 min

*Abbott Radio-Pharmaceuticals, North Chicago, Illinois 60064

(period 1). Draw 5 ml heparinized plasma at midpoint of the time period. Label urine collected at the end of the period and plasma collected at the midpoint.
5. Period 2 (30 min in length): Collect urine at end of period and plasma at midpoint.
6. Period 3 (30 min in length): Collect urine at the end of the period and plasma at the midpoint.
7. Count 1 ml aliquots of urine and plasma samples on scintillation counter with background subtracted.

Calculations

The clearance rates are calculated as follows:

$$C\ ^{125}I = \frac{UV}{P}$$

C = glomerular filtration rate in ml/min
U = urine, cpm/ml ^{125}I
V = urinary flow rate, ml/min
P = plasma, cpm/ml ^{125}I

The average glomerular filtration rate is calculated from the rates for the individual collection periods.

Precautions

The iothalamate clearance test should not be performed on women during pregnancy or lactation or on persons less than 18 years of age.

Interpretation

The normal glomerular filtration rate (GFR) for females is 102–132 ml/min and for males is 110–152 ml/min. This test is mainly valuable as an aid to following the course of renal disease and transplant recipients. In cases of transplant rejection, a rapid GFR determination may be obtained.

The continuous infusion technique is done in a similar method to that of the *p*-aminohippurate clearance (see PAH Clearance).

The single injection technique does not require urine collection and is ideal for pediatric patients or those for whom urine collection is impossible. The glomerular filtration rate is overestimated by about 20% because of the contribution of nonrenal excretory routes (24).

ASSESSING GLOMERULAR FILTRATION RATE BY EVALUATING BLOOD CHEMISTRIES

Assessment of renal function may also be done by measuring plasma concentrations of substances normally excreted by the kidney. In general, one can infer that an elevated concentration of these substances in the plasma is a consequence of the kidneys' decreased capacity for excretion, particularly in regard to the plasma concentration of urea and creatinine.

Urea (blood urea nitrogen or BUN) measurements are the most commonly utilized measurements of renal function. The concentration of urea in the plasma is a reflection of the production of urea (from the dietary intake of protein-containing foodstuffs and the endogenous breakdown of protein) and the excretion of urea by the kidney. Therefore an elevated urea value may come from excessive intake of protein, excessive breakdown of body tissues, or a decreased capacity for excretion by the kidney. The latter is the most common reason for the blood urea nitrogen to be elevated.

Creatinine is a by-product of muscle metabolism. In rare instances, when muscle is damaged, creatinine production may be elevated; hence the concentration of creatinine may rise in the plasma unrelated to any change in renal function. However, in most instances a rise in creatinine concentration reflects a decreased capacity of the kidney to excrete this material. In the older and sometimes debilitated patient who has lost a substantial quantity of body musculature, creatinine production may be greatly diminished, and the plasma concentration of creatinine may appear normal while the actual excretory capacity of the kidney is reduced. That is, the decreased excretory capacity of the kidney is masked by a decreased production of creatinine. Therefore, in most instances, an elevation of the BUN or blood creatinine concentration implies renal dysfunction.

URINE CONCENTRATION

The measurement of renal function may be performed by evaluation of the urine and analysis of its constituents, by analysis of certain constituents of the plasma, and by analysis of simultaneously measured urine and plasma samples. Most simple tests to evaluate renal function include urinalysis. The capacity of the kidney to reabsorb water, one of its important homeostatic mechanisms, is best measured by the maximal concentration of the urine, which can be measured by the specific gravity of the urine or, better and more accurately, by the osmolality of the urine. The reabsorption of water by the kidney is one of its important homeostatic mechanisms. As you will recall, about 150 liters of glomerular filtrate are formed each day while only one liter of urine is ultimately excreted; therefore, 149 liters of glomerular filtrate need to be reabsorbed. Substantial amounts of this fluid are reabsorbed as water alone. As water is removed from the glomerular filtrate, other constituents remaining in the urine are progressively concentrated. As these substances are concentrated, the density of the urine increases (as measured by the specific gravity) and, of course, the concentration of individual molecules increases (as measured by the osmolality of the urine).

URINE CONCENTRATION TEST

The patient is instructed to drink no liquids after 8:00 P.M. the evening preceding the test. (This must be very explicitly stated to the patient.) The test is carried out as follows:

1. At 8:00 A.M. the morning of the test, the patient voids and discards the urine.
2. At 9:00 A.M. and 10:00 A.M., the patient voids and saves the urine sample.
3. These samples are submitted for measurement of osmolality.

The normal individual should have an osmolality of 1000–1200 mOsm/liter.

When water intake is severely restricted and urine specimens do not demonstrate a suitably high specific gravity or osmolality, either renal function is impaired, antidiuretic hormone was not elaborated by the posterior pituitary, or the patient cheated and consumed fluids during the water restriction period. The latter is the most common reason for an abnormal result. Should the patient's physician be concerned about a possible posterior pituitary deficiency of antidiuretic hormones (diabetes insipidus), the test should be repeated with 0.5 cc Vasopressin in oil injected subcutaneously at 2:00 A.M. on the morning of the urine collection. If the urine is not concentrated when collected as in the concentration test, then the kidney function is definitely abnormal and indicates unresponsive antidiuretic hormone.

URINE ACIDIFICATION

Evaluation of the urinary pH may be of assistance in judging functional capacity of the kidney. One of the roles of the kidney is the excretion of excess acid that results from the body's daily metabolism and the intake of an acid diet. The urine then is generally acidic, but fluctuations in the urinary pH occur during the course of the day. However, if the patient has a systemic acidosis, the urine is almost constantly acid if the kidney is acting appropriately. If the urine is not acid (pH less than 6) when the patient has a systemic acidosis, there may be a defect in the kidney which prevents it from adequately excreting acid. This may suggest the diagnosis of renal tubular acidosis, which may be hereditary or acquired. There are numerous disorders that lead to acquired renal tubular acidosis.

TUBULAR REABSORPTION OF GLUCOSE, BICARBONATE, AND PHOSPHATE

The presence of glucose in the urine at a time when the plasma glucose is normal implies that the reabsorptive process for glucose is impaired since normally no glucose is present in the urine until the plasma glucose is distinctly elevated. Such an abnormality suggests a tubular disorder of glucose reabsorption, as found in the Fanconi syndrome or the benign state of renal glycosuria.

Tubular reabsorption is best measured when defects are present in reabsorptive processes. This is most evident when bicarbonate reabsorption or glucose reabsorption is impaired. In these circumstances, bicarbonate or glucose appears in the urine in amounts in excess of what might be anticipated. Bicarbonate serves as an alkalizing substance for urine and, when present in excessive amounts, creates an alkaline urine. While this is not the only substance excreted which creates alkaline urine, an alkaline urine in the presence of acidosis implies an impaired mechanism of bicarbonate reabsorption. Bacterial contamination of the urine may result in ammonia production of sufficient degree to raise the urine pH markedly, but if the urine is sterile and the patient is acidotic, a urinary pH in excess of 6 suggests that the kidney is not handling acid properly and bicarbonate loss is occurring.

A reduced inorganic phosphate concentration in the plasma may be indicative of excessive phosphate loss in the plasma. This occurs in unusual phosphaturic disorders and implies a tubular reabsorptive defect of phosphate. In general, the clearance of phosphate is approximately 10%–15% of the creatinine clearance. When the clearance of phosphate to the clearance of creatinine exceeds this 10%–15% relationship, it implies that excessive phosphaturia is occurring and that there is either a renal defect of phosphate reabsorption or excessive hormonal stimulation to phosphate excretion.

TUBULAR SECRETION

Tubular secretory processes can be measured by the clearance of *p*-aminohippurate (PAH). At low blood levels, PAH may be used to measure renal plasma flow and detect gross deviations from the normal. For example, at a level of 1 mg/dl of plasma, a normal adult excretes 7 mg PAH in 1 min. If 7 mg PAH is excreted per minute, then 700 ml plasma has been cleared of PAH and the renal plasma flow is 700 ml/min.

At high plasma concentrations, 50 mg/dl or more, PAH taxes the tubular excretory mechanism to its maximum. According to Smith (54,55), the rate of maximal excretion by the tubules for such substance transport maximum for PAH (T_m/PAH) is dependent upon the quantity of tubular tissue participating in the excretory process. That is, the test may be used to quantitate the degree of tubular damage in a case of renal impairment. PAH is exclusively secreted unless its concentration exceeds approximately 2 mg/dl.

PAH CLEARANCE (*p*-AMINOHIPPURATE 20%)

The following reagents and equipment are required for PAH clearance testing:

1. Spectrophotometer.
2. *p*-Aminohippurate standard, 1 mg/dl. Free *p*-aminohippuric acid (not the sodium salt which is strongly hygroscopic), 0.90 mg, is dissolved in 100 ml 0.612 M trichloroacetic acid (corresponding to 1 mg sodium salt given in the clearance technique). It is stable indefinitely at room temperature.
3. Sterile saline—30 cc vial.
4. Sodium *p*-aminohippurate 20%—priming and sustaining infusion prepared as follows:
   a. From a 30 cc vial of saline, aspirate 12.5 cc saline and discard.
   b. Add to bottle 12.5 cc PAH 20%.
   c. If a Glofil clearance is to be done, add to this solution 20 microcuries of iothalamate. (This would be approximately 0.1 cc).
   d. Mix the contents thoroughly.
   e. Aspirate the entire contents of the vial into a sterile 30 cc disposable syringe. Place the syringe on a infusion pump.
   f. Inject 0.03 cc/kg into the individual as a priming dose. (This will generally be about 2.2 cc.) Begin the infusion rate at 10 cc/hour. If the patient is estimated to have a decrease in renal function, diminish the rate of the infusion proportionally with the decrease in glomerular filtration rate. For example, if the assumption is that the patient has a glomerular filtration rate of 50% of normal (50 cc/min), then set the infusion rate at 5 cc/hour. If the patient is felt to have 10% of renal function, set the infusion at 1 cc/hour. This step prevents the rate of infusion of PAH from exceeding the renal

excretion of PAH. If PAH is administered too rapidly, as could happen if the rate of infusion were not adjusted, the plasma concentration will progressively increase and exceed the secretory capacity of the renal tubule. At such time one would no longer be measuring renal plasma flow.

5. 0.612 M trichloroacetic acid 10%—100 g trichloroacetic acid (TCA) dissolved in 100 ml distilled water. This is stable indefinitely at room temperature.
6. 0.0145 M sodium nitrite 0.1%—0.1% g sodium nitrite dissolved in 100 ml distilled water. This is stable 1 week if frozen.
7. 3.86 mM N-(1-naphthyl)-ethylenediamine 0.1%—0.1 g dihydrochloride dissolved in 100 ml distilled water. This is stable for 1 month in a dark bottle if frozen. Brown-colored solution should be discarded.
8. Ammonium sulfamate 0.5%—0.5 g ammonium sulfamate dissolved in 100 ml distilled water.
9. Infusion pump (variable speed).
10. Syringes—disposable (5 cc, 30 cc, 50 cc)
11. Urine collection containers—disposable.

PREPARATION OF THE PATIENT

The patient is prepared as follows:

1. Verify that the patient has not recently received any interfering substances such as salicylates, sulfonamides, diuretics, or various contrast media.
2. Patient must be supine and resting quietly either during the morning after a light breakfast or during the afternoon at least 2 hours after lunch.
3. If a bladder catheter is in place, make sure it is draining freely and collect the urine specimen using a syringe to empty the bladder fully. Label "blank." Draw plasma specimen and label "blank."
4. Start IV infusion of PAH and Glofil (if doing simultaneously) as described in step 4 of reagents and equipment.
5. After equilibration of 45 min, have patient empty the bladder totally and begin timed collection period of 30 min. Draw plasma specimen at midpoint. Label as "period 1." Plasma should be spun down as soon as possible after being drawn. Obtain urine at end of 30 min and label "period 1."
6. Proceed as above for Periods 2 and 3, collecting urine and plasma samples at designated times.

PROCEDURE FOR PAH DETERMINATION

PAH determination is made as follows:

1. Deproteinization
   a. Plasma—exactly 0.2 ml added to 1 ml TCA 10%. Mix well, and let stand for 5 min; centrifuge. Dilution is six fold.
   b. Urine—0.02 ml urine diluted with 2 ml TCA 10%. Dilution is 101-fold.
2. Testing. After addition of each reagent, mix well and let stand for 2 min. Color development is complete in 10 min and stable for 1 hour. Read at 540 nm directly on concentration (Table 17–1). Or read absorbance and calculate as follows:

   a. Plasma

   $$\text{mg PAH}/100 \text{ ml} = \frac{\text{O.D. (T)}}{\text{O.D. (S)}_{1 \text{ mg std}}} \times 6.0$$

   b. Urine

   $$\text{mg PAH}/100 \text{ ml} = \frac{\text{O.D. (T)}}{\text{O.D. (S)}_{1 \text{ mg std}}} \times 101$$

   c. Clearance of PAH

   $$C_{\text{PAH}} = \frac{U_{\text{PAH}} \ (\text{mg/dl}) \ V \ (\text{ml/min})}{P_{\text{PAH}} \ (\text{mg/dl})}$$

TABLE 17-1. REAGENT BLANK, STANDARD, AND UNKNOWN TEST TUBES

	Reagent blank	Standard	Unknown
Sodium nitrite, ml	1.0	1.0	1.0
Supernatant, ml			0.5
TCA, ml	0.5		
PAH standard, ml		0.5	
Ammonium sulfamate, ml	1.0	1.0	1.0
N-(1-naphthyl)ethylenediamine, ml	2.5	2.5	2.5

SOURCES OF ERROR

The following are included as possible sources of error.

1. *p*-Aminohippurate penetrates the erythrocytes; therefore, plasma should be used.
2. IV solutions must be administered with caution in patients with low cardiac reserve since a rapid increase in plasma volume can precipitate congestive heart failure.
3. Rapid infusion may cause a sensation of warmth and a sensation of tightness in the patient. In addition, the patient may have the desire to defecate or urinate shortly after administration of priming dose. If this occurs, reduce speed of infusion.
4. Salicylates, sulfonamides, procaine, diuretics, thiazole-sulfone, and various contrast media interfere with analysis and should be withheld for 3 days prior to testing.
5. Patients receiving probenecid will have erroneously low PAH clearance.
6. If no color develops, new sodium nitrite must be prepared. If color develops but fades quickly, prepare new ammonium sulfamate.

INTERPRETATION

Normal values for PAH clearance (corrected for body surface of $1.73 \, M^2$) are for males 675 ± 150 and for females 595 ± 125. This is an excellent and rapid method of renal plasma flow determination.

PART III LABORATORY OPERATION

18 Automation of Urinalysis

The urine specimen is fragile; therefore delays in analysis result in erroneous information. The application of automated techniques to the examination of the urine is only suitable if methods to temporarily delay analysis of the urine are available; at present these methods of temporary preservation are not satisfactory (see Ch. 2, Specimen Collection and Preservation). Urine samples which require rapid analysis appear throughout the 24-hour period at the laboratory, making the utility of automated equipment uncertain except in the larger laboratories with a very high volume.

A bench-top instrument which performs seven chemical tests and gives a value for specific gravity at a sample rate of 120 specimens per hour has been devised.* The system is described by Clemens and Hurtle (16) and is evaluated by Hagar, Brown, and Botero (29). The latter authors compared the performance of the instrumentation to the traditional methods for 2911 specimens and found 98% agreement in terms of positive or negative results. Most of the discrepancies were found to be in highly pigmented urine specimens. The apparent cause of the discrepancies was the effect of the discoloration on the reflectance measurement. The false-positive instrumental results could be avoided by screening the specimens prior to entering them into the automated system.

Automation as a screening procedure in the general population has many possibilities. The detection of renal disease or glucose in the urine is evidenced readily in a screened sample with perhaps only five tests—glucose, protein, ketone, bilirubin, and occult blood.

Semiautomatic equipment can be used for qualitative measurement of certain physical characteristics and chemical constituents of urine. Because of the wide range over which normal urine constituents can vary, it is necessary to run standard samples in order to ensure accuracy. These devices not only speed the quantitative measurement, but the result is generally more precise than hand methods because of the ease of analysis. Such devices include automatic devices for the measurement of osmolality, pH, urine electrolytes, calcium, ammonia, etc.

*Clinilab, Ames Company, Division of Miles Laboratory, Inc., Elkhart, Indiana 46514

19 Quality Control

Quality control plays an important role in accurate urinalysis. Although chemical testing may be ensured to some extent by quality control of reagents, the microscopic examination is almost solely dependent on the technologist's judgment, training, and careful study of the urinary sediment. A number of other nonroutine tests are not quality controlled because commercial products for these procedures are not available. Care must be taken to follow test procedures exactly and to interpret results carefully.

Along with reagents, equipment plays a significant role in routine urinalysis determination. The efficient functioning of these devices must be ensured with control products as well as proper maintenance and operation of the equipment.

Schedules for a quality control program should include the following:

Daily

1. Reading and recording of temperatures for refrigerator and freezer.
2. Checking reagents for quantitating urine sugar (dipstick and reducing).

Weekly

1. Checking all dipstick and tablet test reagents.
2. Inspection of refractometer.
3. Inspection of urinometer.
4. Checking of spectrophotometer for variation from calibration curve.

Semiannually

1. Remaking protein calibration curve for spectrophotometer.
2. Checking glassware for chips, cracks, and contamination.

Annually

1. Reviewing notebook procedures and revising if needed.
2. Checking centrifuge timing
3. Checking thermometer with standard thermometers.

Continually and when indicated

1. Rechecking microscopic and chemical test values not well correlated for possible error (hemoglobin value and microscopic RBCs; protein present with numerous casts).

2. Running of known cystinuric urines when available in parallel with test urine for cystine.
3. Ensuring that reagents are dated on entering the laboratory and used before expiration.
4. Quality controlling reagents of new lot numbers.
5. Storing of quality control products at proper temperatures and using them after reconstitution within expiration dates.
6. Proficiency testing of technologists when possible.
7. Cleaning microscopes and spectrophotometer cuvettes.
8. Maintaining a log book with records of equipment, maintenance, operating instructions, and cautions.

QUALITY CONTROL ACCEPTANCE LIMITS

If a quality control result does not agree with the expected result or value, the technologist should take the following actions:

1. Do not report the results of patient samples analyzed at the same time.
2. Reread the procedure to be sure that the tests were conducted properly.
3. Check instruments to be sure the tests were read at the appropriate wave length, sensitivity, and time, as applicable.
4. Ascertain that reagents were correctly chosen, freshly made, and without signs of deterioration.
5. Verify that the correct calibration curve was employed, if applicable.
6. Verify that the quality control sample was properly chosen, reconstituted, and stored, as applicable.
7. Verify that the lot number and expected result are correct.
8. Correct any inadequacies detected.
9. Obtain a new quality control sample.
10. Repeat all patient samples together with both new and previously used quality control specimens.
11. Compare the results with the expected results. If satisfactory, report the results on the patients; if not, notify the supervisor immediately.

Quality Control for Urine* is an example of a quality control material which provides a convenient, dependable means for monitoring the performance of reagent test strips and other tests commonly used in routine urinalysis. The product is formulated to contain known levels of constituents commonly determined in semiquantitative urinalysis with dipstick procedures when assessing acid–base balance, carbohydrate me-

*General Diagnostics, Division of Warner-Lambert Company, Morris Plains, New Jersey 07950

tabolism, kidney and liver function, etc. Measured values also are listed to provide a means of evaluating the accuracy of analytical procedures often performed on urine specimens. The urine control solutions should retain utility for at least 1 day if they are stored in a tightly stoppered container, refrigerated, and protected from light. This substance provides quality control for tests for blood, bilirubin, glucose, ketones, protein, pH, phenylpyruvate, urobilinogen, red blood cells, and a variety of chemical procedures.

References

1. Addis T: Glomerular Nephritis, Diagnosis and Treatment. New York, Macmillan, 1941, pp 2–3
2. Baird EE: Urinalysis and kidney function. In Race GJ (ed): Laboratory Medicine, Vol 4. Hagerstown, Harper & Row, 1978
3. Baird HW: A reliable paper strip method for the detection of phenylketonuria. J Pediatr 52:715–717, 1958
4. Bates RG: Electrometric pH Determinations. New York, John Wiley & Sons, 1954
5. Bates RG: Concept and determination of pH. In Kolthoff IM, Elving PJ (eds): Treatise on Analytical Chemistry. New York, John Wiley & Sons, 1959, pp 361–404
6. Bates RG: Determination of pH—Theory and Practice. New York, John Wiley & Sons, 1964.
7. Berry HK: Screening for genetic disorders. Fed Proc 34(12):2134–2139, 1975
8. Berry HK, Leonard C, Peters H, Granger M, Chunekamrai N: Detection of metabolic disorders: chromatographic procedures and interpretation of results. Clin Chem 14:1033–1065, 1968
9. Bindel TH, Fennessey PV, Miles BS, Goodman SI: 4–hydroxycyclohexane-1-carboxylic acid: an unusual compound isolated from the urine of children with suspected disorders of metabolism. Clin Chim Acta 66(2):209–217, 1976
10. Bradley GM, Benson ES: Examination of the urine. In Davidsohn I, Henry J (eds): Clinical Diagnosis by Laboratory Methods. Philadelphia, WB Saunders, 1969
11. Bradley MD: Urinary screening tests in the infant and young child. Hum Pathol 2(2):309–320, 1971
12. Brems N: Measurements of pH: electrodes and pertinent apparatus. Acta Anaesthesiol Scand (11):199, 1962
12a. Brenner BM, Rector FC (ed): The Kidney. Philadelphia, WB Saunders, 1976, pp 318–343
13. Cartwright GE: Diagnostic Laboratory Hematology, 4th ed. New York, Grune & Stratton, 1968
14. Chemstrip Manufacturer's Instructions. Bio-Dynamics/bmc, Division of Boehringer Mannheim, Indianapolis, IN 46250
15. Cheronis ND: Micro and Semimicro Methods. New York, Interscience Publishers, 1954, p 452
16. Clemens AH, Hurtle RL: Automatic system for urine analysis. I. System design and development. Clin Chem 18:789–793, 1972
17. Court JM, Davies HE, Ferguson R: Diastix and Ketodiastix, a new semiquantitative test for glucose in urine. Med J Aust 1:525–528, 1972
18. DeAngelis GG: Testing for drugs. II. Techniques and issues. Int J Addict 8(6):997–1014, 1973
19. D'Eramo EM, McAnear JT: The significance of urinalysis in treatment of hospitalized dental patients. Oral Surg 38:36–41, 1974
20. Drabkin DL: The normal pigment of urine: the relationship of urinary pigment output to diet and metabolism. J Biol Chem 75:443–479, 1927
21. Drabkin DL: The normal pigment of the urine: a new method for its extraction. J Biol Chem 88:433–442, 1930

22. Effersoe P, Tidstrom B: Detection of myeloma protein in urine by a new quick method. J Lab Clin Med 50:134–138, 1957
23. Efron ML: Aminoaciduria. N Engl J Med 272:1058–1067, 1965
24. Emmet M, White MG: Personal communication
25. Feigl F: Spot Tests in Inorganic Analysis, 5th ed. New York, Elsevier, 1958
26. Frimpter GW: Aminoacidurias due to inherited disorders of metabolism. N Engl J Med 289:835–841; 895–901, 1973
27. Garrod AE: Inborn Errors of Metabolism, 2nd ed. London, Oxford Medical Publications, 1923
28. Haber F, Klemensiewicz Z: Über elektrische phasengrenzkräfte. Z Physik Chem 67:385, 1909
29. Hager CB, Brown JR, Botero JM: Automatic system for urine analysis. II. Evaluation of the system. Clin Chem 18:794–799, 1972
30. Henry RJ, Cannon DC, Winkelman JW: Clinical Chemistry, Principles and Technics, 2nd ed. Hagerstown, Harper & Row, 1974
31. Herman JR: Urology, A View Through the Retrospectroscope. Hagerstown, Harper & Row, 1973
32. Hughes WS: The potential difference between glass and electrolytes in contact with the glass. J Am Chem Soc 44:2860, 1922
33. Keele KD: The Evolution of Clinical Methods in Medicine. Springfield, IL, CC Thomas, 1963
34. Kerridge PT: The use of the glass electrode in biochemistry. Biochem J 19:611, 1925
35. Kilduffe RA: Clinical Urinalysis and Its Interpretation. Philadelphia, FA Davis, 1937
36. King SE, Gronbeck C: Benign and pathologic albuminuria: a study of 600 hospitalized cases. Ann Intern Med 36:765–785, 1952
37. Leach CS, Rambault PC, Fischer CL: A comparative study of two methods of urine preservation. Clin Biochem 8(2):108–117, 1975
38. Major RH: Classic Descriptions of Disease. Springfield, IL, CC Thomas, 1932
39. Manuel Y, Revillard JP, Betuel H (eds): Proteins in Normal and Pathological Urine. Baltimore, University Park Press, 1970
40. Marsh JB, Drabkin DL: Kidney phosphatases in alimentary hyperglycemia and phlorhizin glycosuria: a dynamic mechanism for renal threshold for glucose. J Biol Chem 168:61–73, 1947
41. Miller SE (ed): A Textbook of Clinical Pathology, 5th ed. Baltimore, Williams & Wilkins, 1955
42. Mitchell CB: pH and acid-base disturbances. In Race GJ (ed): Laboratory Medicine, Vol 1. Hagerstown, Harper & Row, 1978
43. Ostow M, Philo S: The chief urinary pigment: the relationship between the rate of excretion of the yellow urinary pigment and the metabolic rate. Am J Med Sci 207:507–512, 1944.
44. Perry TL, Hansen S, MacDougall L: Urinary screening test in the prevention of mental deficiency. Can Med Assoc J 95:89–95, 1966
45. Pesce AJ: Methods used for the analysis of proteins in the urine. Nephron 13(1)93–104, 1974
46. Pictoclinic: Detection of Phenylketonuria, Vol 2, No. 6. Elkhart, IN, Ames Company, 1964
47. Ragsdale N, Koch R: Phenylketonuria: detection and therapy. Am J Nurs 64:90–96, 1964

48. Richards AN: Processes of urine formation. Proc R Soc Med 26:398–432, 1938
49. Ritzmann SE, Thurm RH, Levin WC: Alpha-2-myelomasthe fallibility of arbitrary classifications of myeloma proteins. Tex Rep Biol Med 21:7492, 1963
50. Seegmiller JE, Zannoni, VG, Laster L, LaDu BN: An enzymatic spectrophotometric method for the determination of homogentisic acid in plasma and urine. J Biol Chem 236:774–777, 1961
51. Shih VE: Laboratory Techniques for the Detection of Hereditary Metabolic Disorders. Cleveland, CRC Press (Division of the Chemical Rubber Company), 1973
52. Siggard-Andersen O: Titratable acid or base of body fluids. Ann NY Acad Sci 133:41–58, 1966.
53. Sills JL: Urinalysis Notebook, unpublished manual prepared in Urinalysis Section, Baylor University Medical Center, Dallas, TX, 1975
54. Smith HW: Lectures on the kidney. In The William Henry Welch Lectures. Lawrence, KN, University Extension Division, University of Kansas, 1943
55. Smith HW: The Kidney Structure and Function in Health and Disease. New York, Oxford University Press, 1951
56. Sommerfelt SC, Hoveid P, Wynstroot E: The excretion of homogentisic acid, phenylalamine and tyrosine in an alkaptonuric subject. Acta Med Scand 170:51–58, 1961
57. Spaeth GL, Barber GW: Prevalence of homocystinuria among the mentally retarded: evaluation of a specific screening test. Pediatrics 40:586–589, 1967
58. Stadie WC: An electron tube potentiometer for the determination of pH with the glass electrode. J Biol Chem 83:477, 1929
59. Sternheimer R: A supravital cytodiagnostic stain for urinary sediments. JAMA 231(8):826–832, 1975
60. Sun MW, Stein E, Gruen FW: A single column method for determination of urinary delta aminolevulinic acid. Clin Chem 15:183–189, 1969.
61. Thomas GH, Howell RR: Selected Screening Tests for Genetic Metabolic Diseases. Chicago, Year Book Medical, 1973
62. Tietz NW (ed): Fundamentals of Clinical Chemistry, 2nd ed. Philadelphia, WB Saunders, 1976
63. Watson CJ, Schwartz S: A simple test for urinary porphobilinogen. Proc Soc Exp Biol Med 47:393–394, 1941
64. Wells BB: Clinical Pathology: Application and Interpretation. Philadelphia, WB Saunders, 1950
65. Wilkerson HLC, Krall LP: Diabetes in a New England town: a study of 3,516 persons in Oxford, Massachusetts. JAMA 135:209–216, 1947
66. Wilson DM: Urinalysis and other tests of renal function. Minn Med 58(1):9–17, 1975
67. Young DS, Pestaner LC, Gibberman V: Effects of drugs on clinical laboratory tests. Clin Chem 21(5):1D–432D, 1975

GENERAL REFERENCES

Lippman RW: Urine and the Urinary Sediment, 2nd ed. Springfield, IL, CC Thomas, 1973

Pitts RF: Physiology, Kidney and Body Fluids, 3rd ed. Chicago, Yearbook Medical, 1974

Spencer ES, Pederson I: Hand Atlas of the Urinary Sediment, 2nd ed. Baltimore, University Park Press, 1976

Urine Under the Microscope. Nutley, NJ, ROCOM Press, Division of Hoffmann-LaRoche, 1973

INDEX

Abuse of drugs, screening for, 86
Acetoacetic acid in urine, tests for, 34–37
Acetone in urine, tests for, 34–37
Acid
  boric, for specimen preservation, 10
  and heat test in measurement of protein in urine, 40
Acid urine, crystals in, 22–23
Acidification, urine, in evaluation of renal function, 95–96
Addis count, 48–50
Albustix, purpose and technique of, 28
Alkaline urine, crystals in, 23
Alkaptonuria, screening for, 75–76
Amino acids
  metabolism of, disorders of, screening for, 68–69
  pediatric screening for, 84
  transport of, disorders of, screening for, 70
Aminoacidurias, screening for, 68–75
p-Aminohippurate (PAH), clearance of, in evaluation
  of renal function, 97–100
    interpretation of, 100
    preparation of patient for, 98
    procedure for, 99
    sources of error in, 100
  of tubular secretion, 96–97
β-Aminoisobutyricaciduria, screening for, 78
Ammonia biurate crystals in urine, 23
Amorphous phosphates
  cloudiness of urine due to, 12–13
  crystals of, in urine, 23
Amorphous urates
  crystals of, in urine, 23, 24
  effect of, on urine, 13
Aniline phthalate, preparation and use of, 74
p-Anisidine, preparation and use of, 73
Antidiuretic hormone (ADH) in control of water removal from urine, 14
Automation of urinalysis, 101

Bacteria in microscopic examination of urine, 21–22

Bacterial casts in urine, 25
Bacteriuria, pediatric screening for, 82
Bence-Jones protein in urine, 45–48
Benzidine test for blood, 52
Benzoate-Urotropin tablet for specimen preservation, 10
Bicarbonate, tubular reabsorption of, in evaluation of renal function, 96–97
Bile in urine, 53–55
Bili-labstix, purpose and technique of, 28
Bilirubin in urine, 53–55
Bilirubinuria, 54
Biuret method in measurement of protein in urine, 42
Bladder
  catheterization of, in-and-out, 8
  suprapubic aspiration of, 8–9
Blood
  filtration of, in kidney, 3
  urine, benzidine or orthotoluidine test for, 52
Blood chemistries, evaluation of, assessment of glomerular filtration rate by, 94
Boric acid for specimen preservation, 10
Bromcresol green, preparation and use of, 73

Calcium in urine, 65–66
Calcium carbonate crystals in urine, 23
Calcium oxalate crystals in urine, 23
Calcium phosphate crystals in urine, 23
Calculus, renal, analysis of, 65
Carotene in urine, 63
Casts
  in microscopic examination of urine, 24-26
  structures mistaken for, 26–27
Catheter specimen, method of collection of, 8
Catheterization of bladder, in-and-out, 8
Cells, epithelial, in microscopic examination of urine, 21
Chemical screening in infants, 83
Chemstrip 8, purpose and technique of, 28
Children, screening of, for disease, 82–86
Chloroform for specimen preservation, 10

Index

Clarity of urine, 12–14
Clinical screening, urinalysis for, 27–29
Clinitest, purpose and technique of, 29
Color of urine, 12, 13
Combistix, purpose and technique of, 28
Combustix in measurement of protein in urine, 42
Copper-reducing substance, pediatric surgery for, 83
Coproporphyrin in urine, 61
Creatinine clearance
   short-term, in measurement of glomerular filtration rate, 91–92
   twenty-four hour, in measurement of glomerular filtration rate, 91
Crystals
   in microscopic examination of urine, 22–24
   minute, differentiation of, from casts, 26
Cystathioninuria, screening for, 78
Cystine crystals in urine, 23–24
Cystinuria, screening for, 76–77
Cytodiagnostic stain, supravital, for urinary sediments, 27

Diabetic acid in urine, tests for, 34–37
Diastix, purpose and technique of, 29
Diazotized sulfanilic acid, preparation and use of, 73
Dichloroquinonechlorimide, preparation and use of, 74
p-Dimethylaminobenzaldehyde, preparation and use of, 74
p-Dimethylaminocinnamaldehyde, preparation and use of, 74
Dip tests for carbohydrate excretion disorders, 71, 72
Dipstick method
   for bilirubin detection, 54–55
   for urobilinogen detection, 56–57
Disease, pediatric screening for, 82–86
Drug abuse, screening for, 86
Drying, vacuum, for specimen preservation, 10–11
Dye binding in measurement of protein in urine, 42

Epithelial cells in microscopic examination of urine, 21

Erythrocytes in microscopic examination of urine, 20–21
Erythropoietic porphyria, 59–60

Fat in urine, 64
Fat bodies, oval, differentiation of, from casts, 26
Fatty casts in urine, 25
Ferricyanide-nitroprusside, preparation and use of, 73
Foam in urine, 14
Folin-Lowry method in measurement of protein in urine, 42
Formalin for specimen preservation, 10
Freezing for specimen preservation, 10-11
Fungi in microscopic examination of urine, 22

"Glitter" cells in microscopic examination of urine, 19
Glomerular filtration rate
   assessment of, by evaluating blood chemistries, 94
   measurement of, 89–93
      iothalamate clearance in, 92–93
      short-term creatinine clearance in, 91–92
      twenty-four hour creatinine clearance in, 91
Glomerular proteinuria, causes of, 38
Glucose
   tubular reabsorption of, in evaluation of renal function, 96–97
   in urine, 31–34
      measurement of, 32–34
Glucose oxidase testing for glucose, 33
Glycinuria, screening for, 77
Granular casts in urine, 24–25
Gravity, specific. *See* Specific gravity of urine
Guthrie test for phenylketonuria, 81

Harrison spot test for bilirubin detection, 54

Heat and acid test in measurement of protein in urine, 40, 42
Hemacombistix, purpose and technique of, 28
Hemastix, purpose and technique of, 28
Hematuria, causes of, 20–21
Hemoglobinuria, 51–53
  hemolytic infections and, 52–53
Hemolytic infections and hemoglobinuria, 52–53
Hemosiderin in urine, Rous test for, 53
Histidinemia, screening for, 77
Homocystinuria, screening for, 78, 79
Hormone, antidiuretic, in control of water removal from urine, 14
Hyaline casts in urine, 24
Hydrogen concentration of urine, measurement of, 30–31
Hydrometer for testing specific gravity, 16
Hyperosthenuria, definition of, 15
Hyperoxaluria, screening for, 77
Hyperprolinemia, screening for, 78
Hypervalinemia, screening for, 77
Hyposthenuria, definition of, 15

Ictostix, purpose and technique of, 28
Ictotest for bilirubin detection, 55
Inborn errors of metabolism, 67–82
Infants, screening of
  for phenylketonuria, 80–81
  for tyrosinosis, 81
Infections, hemolytic, and hemoglobinuria, 52–53
Iodine-azide, preparation and use of, 74
Iothalamate clearance in measurement of glomerular filtration rate, 92–93
Isatin, preparation and use of, 73
Isosthenuria, definition of, 15

Joseph's syndrome, screening for, 78

Keto-diastix, purpose and technique of, 29
Ketone bodies in urine, 34–37
  tests for
    principle of, 35

Ketone bodies in urine, tests for (*continued*)
  reagent strips for, 36–37
  techniques of, 35–36
  verification test of, 36
Ketostix, purpose and technique of, 29
Kidneys
  function of, 2–5
    tests, 87–100. *See also* Renal function tests
  tissue from, in urine, 26
Kingsbury-Clark method in measurement of protein in urine, 41, 43
Kjeldahl method in measurement of protein in urine, 42

Laboratory operation, 101–104
Labstix, purpose and technique of, 28
Lange's method of testing for acetone or acetoacetic acid, 35–36, 37
Lead poisoning, pediatric screening for, 84
Leukocytes in microscopic examination of urine, 18–20

Maple syrup urine disease, screening for, 78, 80
Melanin in urine, 62–63
Metabolic derangements, generalized, 67–82
Metabolism, inborn errors of, 67–82
Methanamine for specimen preservation, 10
Microscopic examination of urine, 18–27
  findings and interpretation of, 18–27
  method of, 18
Microstix, purpose and techniques of, 28
Midstream urine, method of collection of, 7–8
Mucopolysaccharides, excessive, pediatric screening for, 84
Mucous threads, differentiation of, from casts, 26
Multistix reagent strips, purpose and technique of, 28
Myoglobin in urine, 50–51

Naphthoresorcinol, preparation and use of, 74
Neonates, screening of
　for phenylketonuria, 80–81
　for tyrosinosis, 81
Ninhydrin, preparation and use of, 73
Nitroprusside test for ketone bodies in urine, 34–37

Odor of urine, 14
Orthostatic proteinuria, 43–44
Orthotoluidine test for blood, 52
Osmolality of urine, 14–17

Parasites in microscopic examination of urine, 22
Pediatric screening for disease, 82–86
pH, urinary, 30–31
　in evaluation of renal function, 95–96
Phenistix, purpose and technique of, 29
Phenylketonuria, screening for, 80–81
Phosphates
　amorphous
　　cloudiness of urine due to, 12–13
　　crystals of, in urine, 23
　calcium, crystals of, in urine, 23
　masses of, differentiation of, from casts, 26
　triple, crystals of, in urine, 23
　tubular reabsorption of, in evaluation of renal function, 96–97
Pigmented casts in urine, 25
Pigments, urinary, 50–64
Poisoning, lead, pediatric screening for, 84
Porphobilinogen in urine, 57–62
Porphyria
　acute intermittent, 60
　erythropoietic, 59–60
Porphyria cutanea tarda, 60
Porphyrins in urine, 57–62
Porphyrinuria, 58–59
Precipitation methods in measurement of protein in urine, 41–43
Preservation of specimen, 9–11
Protein in urine, 37–48
　Bence-Jones, 45–48

Protein in urine (*continued*)
　measurement of, 39–41
　　interferences and false tests in, 44
　　spectrophotometer curve for, preparation of, 45
Proteinuria
　Bence-Jones, detection of, 45–48
　glomerular, causes of, 38
　mechanism of, 37-39
　orthostatic, 43–44
　tubular, differential diagnosis of, 38–39

Quality control in urinalysis, 102–104

Reagent strip test in measurement of protein in urine, 40–41
Reagent strips for ketone testing, 36–37
Reagents for screening for metabolic disorders, 73–75
Red blood cell casts in urine, 25
Refractive index in measurement of protein in urine, 42
Refractometer for testing specific gravity, 16
Refrigeration for specimen preservation, 10
Renal calculus, analysis of, 66
Renal function tests, 87–100
　of glomerular filtration, 89–94
　physiologic basis for, 87–89
　of tubular reabsortion of glucose bicarbonate and phosphate, 96–97
　of urine concentration, 94–96
Rothera's method of testing for acetone or acetoacetic acid, 37
Rous test for hemosiderin, 53

Screening, clinical, urinalysis for, 27–29
Screening tests for metabolic derangements, 67–82
Sediments
　pediatric screening for, 83
　telescoped, in microscopic examination of urine, 26

Index

Sediments (*continued*)
urinary, spuravital cytodiagnostic stain for, 27
Semiautomated device for testing specific gravity, 16
Specific gravity of urine, 14–17
in measurement of protein in urine, 42
methods of testing, 16
pediatric screening for, 83
Specimen
collection methods for, 7–9
handling of, 9
preservation of, 9–11
Spectrophotometer curve for protein in urine, preparation of, 45
Spot plate tests for carbohydrates excretion disorders, 71, 72
Stain, cytodiagnostic, supravital, for urinary sediments, 27
Stones, renal, analysis of, 66
Sugar spot tests for carbohydrates excretion disorders, 71, 72
Sugars in urine, 31–34
measurement of, 32–34
Sulfanilic acid, preparation and use of, 73
Sulfosalicylic acid test in measurement of protein in urine, 40
Supernatant, pediatric screening for, 84
Supine urine in detection of orthostatic proteinuria, 44
Suprapubic aspiration of bladder, 8–9
Supravital cytodiagnostic stain for urinary sediments, 27

Telescoped sediment in microscopic examination of urine, 26
Testape, purpose and technique of, 29
Thiamine in urine, 63
Three-glass urine, method of collection of, 7
Tissue, renal, in urine, 26
Toluene for specimen preservation, 10
Toluene sulfonic acid screening test for Bence-Jones protein, 47–48
Toluidine blue, preparation and use of, 73
Triple phosphate crystals in urine, 23
Tubular proteinuria, differential diagnosis of, 38–39

Tubular reabsorption of glucose, bicarbonate, and phosphate in evaluation of renal function, 96–97
Tyrosinosis, screening for, 81

Upright urine in detection of orthostatic proteinuria, 44
Urates
amorphous
crystals of, in urine, 23, 24
effect of, on urine, 13
masses of, differentiation of, from casts, 26
Ureteral sample, method of collection of, 8
Ureteroileostomy sample, method of collection of, 8
Uric acid crystals in urine, 23, 24
Urinalysis
automation of, 101
history of, 1–2
laboratory for, operation of, 101–104
purpose of, 5–6
quality control for, 102–104
routine
observation in, 6
significance of, 2–5
testing procedures in, 12–100
Urinary pigments, 50–64
Urinary sediments, supravital cytodiagnostic stain for, 27
Urine
acid, crystals in, 22–23
Addis count in, 48–50
alkaline, crystals in, 23
calcium in, 65–66
clarity of, 12–14
color of, 12, 13
concentration of, in evaluation of renal function, 94–96
constituents of, 2–3, 4–5
fat in, 64
foam in, 14
glucose and other sugars in, 31–34
ketones in, 34–37
metabolic derangements in, generalized, 67–82
microscopic examination of, 18–27
midstream, method of collection of, 7–8
odor of, 14

Urine (*continued*)
  osmolality of, 17
  output of, average daily, 5
  pH of, 30–31
    in evaluation of renal function, 95–96
  physical characteristics of, 12–14
  pigments in, 50–64
  protein in, 37–48
  renal tissue in, 26
  screening of
    clinical, 27–29
    for diseases, drugs, or poisons, 82–86
  specific gravity of, 14–16. *See also*
    Specific gravity of urine
  specimen of. *See* Specimen
  supine, in detection of orthostatic proteinuria, 44
  three-glass, method of collection of, 7
  upright, in detection of orthostatic proteinuria, 44
Urinometer for testing specific gravity, 16
Uristix, purpose and technique of, 28
Urobilinogen in urine, 55–57
  methods for detection of, 56–57
Urobilinogenuria, 55–56
Urobilinuria, 55–56
Urobilistix, purpose and technique of, 28

Vacuum drying for specimen preservation, 10–11
Vitamin A in urine, 63
Vitamin B₁ in urine, 63
Voided sample, method of collection of, 7

Watson's test for porphyrin, 62
Watson-Schwartz test for porphobilinogen, 61–62
Waxy casts in urine, 24
White blood cell casts in urine, 25

Xanthine crystals in urine, 24

Yeast cells, differentiation of, from erythrocytes in urine, 20, 21

Veterans Administration Hospital
Laboratory Service (113)
Lexington, Kentucky 40507